ELECTRO-CARDIOGRAPHY
SELF–ASSESSMENT

Edward K. Chung, M.D., F.A.C.P., F.A.C.C.
Professor of Medicine
Jefferson Medical College of
Thomas Jefferson University

Director of the Heart Station and
Attending Physician (Cardiologist)
Thomas Jefferson University Hospital
Philadelphia, Pennsylvania

APPLETON & LANGE
Norwalk, Connecticut/San Mateo, California

0-8385-2168-1

88 89 90 91 92 / 10 9 8 7 6 5 4 3 2 1

Prentice-Hall of Australia, Pty. Ltd., Sydney
Prentice-Hall Canada, Inc.
Prentice-Hall Hispanoamericana, S.A., Mexico
Prentice-Hall of India Private Limited, New Delhi
Prentice-Hall International (UK) Limited, London
Prentice-Hall of Japan, Inc., Tokyo
Prentice-Hall of Southeast Asia (Pte.) Ltd., Singapore
Whitehall Books Ltd., Wellington, New Zealand
Editora Prentice-Hall do Brasil Ltda., Rio de Janeiro

Chung, Edward K.
    Electrocardiography : self-assessment / Edward K. Chung.
        p. cm.
    Bibliography: p.
    Includes index.
    ISBN 0-8385-2168-1
    1. Electrocardiography—Examinations, questions, etc.
2. Arrhythmia—Treatment—Examinations, questions, etc.   I. Chung,
Edward K. Electrocardiography, practical applications with
vectorial principles.   II. Title.
    [DNLM: 1. Electrocardiography—case studies.   WG 140 C559eb]
RC683.5.E5C4632 1988
616.1′207547—dc19
DNLM/DLC
for Library of Congress   87-35168
                                                              CIP

Production Editor: Mary Beth Miller
Designer: Kathleen Peters Ceconi

PRINTED IN THE UNITED STATES OF AMERICA

To
My Wife, Lisa
and
To Our Children, Linda and Christopher

CONTENTS

PREFACE

This book, *Electrocardiography: Self-Assessment*, includes 200 cases of common cardiac abnormalities and arrhythmias that are frequently encountered in our medical practice.

Each case describes a short case history to aid in the interpretation of the ECG tracing. The reverse side of each page gives a full analysis of the interpretation of the tracing so that the reader can assess his or her ECG diagnosis. In the majority of cases three simultaneous ECG leads (leads V_1, II, and V_5), recorded by three-channel ECG equipment, are shown for the accurate diagnosis. In addition to the ECG diagnosis, the pertinent clinical significance and the therapeutic approach are included in many instances.

The arrangement of the text and illustrations is based upon the author's experience in teaching medical students, house staff, cardiology fellows, cardiac care nurses, and physicians with various backgrounds.

The unique feature of this book, like all other books by the author, is a practical approach with its clinical applications that will directly assist each reader in the diagnosis and management of his or her patient. The author hopes that the book will be of particular value to all primary care physicians including cardiologists, internists, family physicians, and emergency room physicians, in addition to medical house staff and cardiology fellows. Medical students, cardiac care nurses, and physicians with other specialties (eg, anesthesiologists, cardiovascular surgeons), of course, will learn about various common ECG abnormalities and cardiac arrhythmias in detail by reading this book.

The secretarial duties were carried out cheerfully by Carole Pyzia, the author's personal secretary. Her valuable contribution is greatly appreciated. It has been my pleasure to work with the staff of the publisher, Appleton & Lange.

Lastly, I will always be deeply grateful to and appreciative of my father, Il-Chun Chung, M.D., who has always offered guidance and inspiration.

Edward K. Chung, M.D.
Bryn Mawr, Pennsylvania

ABBREVIATIONS

AF. Atrial fibrillation

APC. Atrial premature contraction

ASD. Atrial septal defect

AT. Atrial tachycardia

A-V. Atrioventricular

A-V JEB. A-V junctional escape beat

A-V JER. A-V junctional escape rhythm

A-V JPC. A-V junctional premature contraction

A-V JT. A-V junctional tachycardia

BBBB. Bilateral bundle branch block

BFB. Bifascicular block

BP. Blood pressure

BTS. Bradytachyarrhythmia syndrome

CABS. Coronary artery bypass surgery

CAD. Coronary artery disease

CCU. Coronary care unit

CHF. Congestive heart failure

CNS disorders. Central nervous system disorders

COPD. Chronic obstructive pulmonary disease

CPR. Cardiopulmonary resuscitation

CSS. Carotid sinus stimulation

DC shock. Direct current shock

DI. Digitalis intoxication

ECG. Electrocardiogram

EPS. Electrophysiologic study

ER. Emergency room

IHSS. Idiopathic hypertrophic subaortic stenosis

JEB. Junctional escape beats

JER. Junctional escape rhythm

JPC. Junctional premature contraction

JT. Junctional tachycardia

LAH. Left atrial hypertrophy

LBBB. Left bundle branch block

LGL syndrome. Lown-Ganong-Levine syndrome

LVH. Left ventricular hypertrophy

MAT. Multifocal atrial tachycardia

MI. Myocardial infarction

MVPS. Mitral valve prolapse syndrome

PAT. Paroxysmal atrial tachycardia

PTCA. Percutaneous transluminal coronary angioplasty

RAH. Right atrial hypertrophy

RBBB. Right bundle branch block

RHD. Rheumatic heart disease

RVH. Right ventricular hypertrophy

S-A. Sinoatrial

SSS. Sick sinus syndrome

TFB. Trifascicular block

V-A. Ventriculoatrial

VEB. Ventricular escape beat

VER. Ventricular escape rhythm

VF. Ventricular fibrillation

VPC. Ventricular premature contraction

VT. Ventricular tachycardia

WPW syndrome. Wolff-Parkinson-White syndrome

CHAPTER ONE

MYOCARDIAL ISCHEMIA, INJURY, AND INFARCTION

CASE 1

A 57-year-old woman was admitted to CCU because of chest pain. She was *not* taking any medication before this admission.

1. What is the ECG diagnosis?

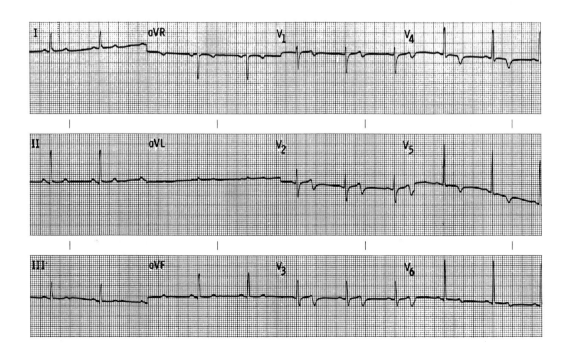

Diagnosis

The cardiac rhythm is sinus, with a rate of 60 beats per minute. Obviously, the T waves are inverted in leads V_{1-6}, indicative of anterior myocardial ischemia. Thus the clinical diagnosis of angina pectoris was entertained.

It should be noted that the resting ECG may be entirely normal in patients with angina pectoris (50–75 percent of cases). Under this circumstance myocardial ischemia can be readily induced by an exercise (treadmill) ECG test when there is significant coronary artery lesion. It has been shown that the exercise ECG test result is markedly abnormal (positive test) in up to 90–100 percent of cases when there is triple-vessel disease or left main coronary artery lesion. By and large, 70 percent or more narrowing of the coronary artery is considered to be a significant coronary artery stenosis. When there is only a single vessel CAD, the exercise ECG test result is often negative (up to 50 percent of cases).

Myocardial ischemia may be manifested on the ECG by tall T waves (subendocardial ischemia), inverted T waves (subepicardial ischemia), depression of ST segment (subendocardial injury), or elevation of ST segment (subepicardial injury).

It is a general trend to perform further studies such as coronary arteriography to determine the precise coronary artery anatomy so that proper therapeutic approach can be chosen (eg, coronary angioplasty, CABS) in patients with CAD, especially when the patient is symptomatic.

A 55-year-old man was admitted to the CCU because of recurrent chest pain via ER. Several ECG tracings were obtained from this patient in his physician's office prior to admission, but all ECGs were said to be within normal limits.

1. What is the ECG diagnosis?
2. What is most likely the clinical diagnosis?
3. What is the proper way to handle this patient?

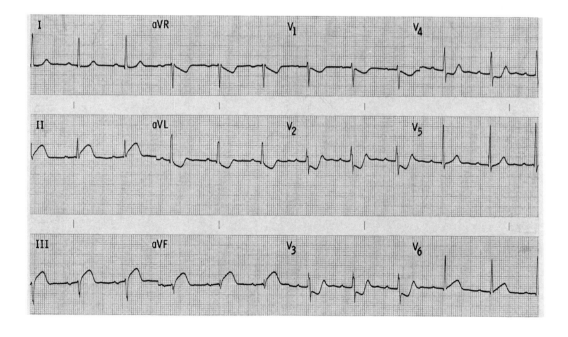

Diagnosis

The underlying cardiac rhythm is sinus (rate:65 beats per minute) with first degree A-V block.

The ST segment is elevated in leads II, III, aVF, and V_6, and the ST segment is depressed in leads V_{1-4}. These ECG findings are indicative of diaphragmatic (inferior)-posterolateral subepicardial injury. This patient was closely monitored in the CCU, and the above-mentioned ST segment changes only occurred while he was having chest pain. Otherwise his ECG always returned to normal.

The diagnosis of coronary artery spasm was entertained without much difficulty, and the patient never developed abnormal Q waves diagnostic of MI. Likewise, serum enzymes failed to rise in this patient. His chest pain was eliminated completely when nifedipine was administered (10 mg every six hours). The diagnosis of acute MI was excluded.

It has been shown that some patients with coronary artery spasm may have fixed coronary artery lesion(s) (up to 50 percent of cases in some reports). Therefore it is advisable to perform coronary arteriography so that CABS or PTCA can be performed in selected patients with coexisting fixed coronary artery lesion(s), especially when medical therapy alone is not fully effective.

At times various provocative tests (eg, ergonovine maleate) may be performed to induce coronary artery spasm when the ECG findings and the clinical history are equivocal. When one of the channel blockers is ineffective, other calcium channel blockers may be tried in patients with coronary artery spasm. Calcium channel blockers are also very effective in the prevention and treatment of various arrhythmias associated with coronary artery spasm. The spasm may involve only one coronary artery segment, but multiple locations may be involved diffusely.

CASE 3

A 73-year-old woman with previous history of a heart attack underwent CABS, and her postoperative course was uneventful. This ECG tracing was obtained a few hours after CABS.

1. What is the ECG diagnosis?
2. What is the proper therapeutic approach?

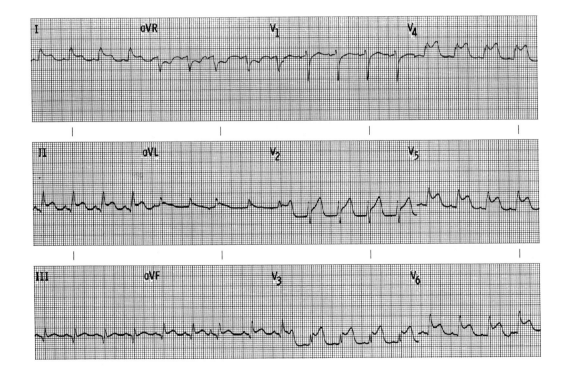

Diagnosis

The cardiac rhythm is sinus, with a rate of 100 beats per minute. Note an APC on the seventh beat.

It is obvious to recognize that the ST segment is diffusely elevated in many leads, and this ECG finding represents acute pericarditis secondary to CABS. In a broad sense surgery-induced pericarditis is a form of postcardiotomy syndrome (postpericardiotomy syndrome). It can be said that open-heart–surgery-induced pericarditis is probably the commonest form of acute pericarditis when dealing with patients who are treated in the all teaching hospitals (eg, university hospitals) with very active cardiovascular service.

Another ECG abnormality is abnormal Q waves in leads II, III, and aVF, indicative of diaphragmatic (inferior) MI.

In most cases surgery-induced pericarditis is a transient phenomenon and is self-limited. No active treatment is necessary under this circumstance.

CASE 4

This ECG tracing was obtained from a 50-year-old man with a recent heart attack. He was admitted to the CCU, and his post-MI course was uneventful.

    1. What is the ECG diagnosis?

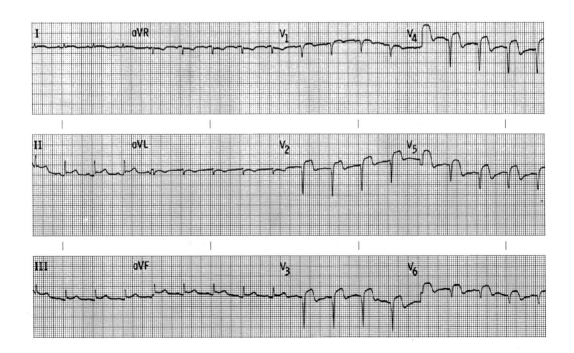

Diagnosis

The underlying cardiac rhythm is sinus, with a rate of 100 beats per minute. Acute extensive anterior MI is diagnosed without any difficulty on the basis of QS waves in all precordial leads (leads V_{1-6}) associated with ST segment elevation and T wave inversion. When MI becomes a few days to one week old, the ST segment returns to isoelectric line, but the T wave inversion may last much longer. At times the T wave inversion may last many weeks, months, or even indefinitely without any particular reason.

Ventricular aneurysm is strongly considered when the ST segment elevation persists more than 1 week after an acute MI, particularly when MI is massive in the anterior wall of the left ventricle, as in this patient.

The term "low voltage" is used when the QRS amplitude in the limb leads is markedly diminished. In particular, the low voltage is diagnosed on the ECG when the sum of the QRS amplitude (both upright and downward combined) in leads I, II, and III is 15 mm or less, as seen in this case. Low voltage is a relatively common ECG finding in patients with acute MI, advanced CHF, cardiogenic shock, and cardiomyopathy. Other causes of low voltage include COPD, myxedema, marked obesity, advanced age, pericardial effusion, constrictive pericarditis, pleural effusion, and massive pneumothorax.

This ECG tracing was taken in the CCU from a 46-year-old man with CAD. He was relatively comfortable except for intermittent, mild chest pain, with no significant hemodynamic abnormality.

1. What is the cardiac rhythm diagnosis?

2. What is the most likely cause of his arrhythmia?

3. What is the proper therapeutic approach to this arrhythmia?

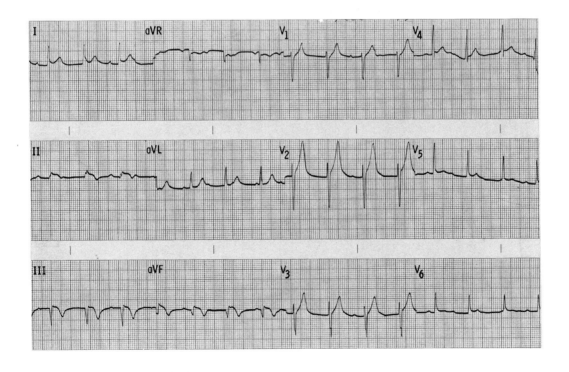

Diagnosis

Some inexperienced readers may misdiagnose as normal sinus rhythm by assuming that every sinus P wave is conducted to the ventricles. However, most experienced readers should be able to recognize that the atrial and the ventricular activities are independent throughout the tracing. Namely, the correct cardiac rhythm diagnosis is sinus tachycardia (atrial rate: 120 beats per minute) with nonparoxysmal A-V JT (A-V JT, rate: 81 beats per minute), producing complete A-V dissociation. It should be noted that the atrial (sinus) cycle is regular, and the ventricular cycle is also regular, but there is no relationship between the P waves and the QRS complexes, meaning complete A-V dissociation.

The direct cause of this nonparoxysmal A-V junctional tachycardia is impairment of blood supply to the A-V junction secondary to right coronary artery stenosis or occlusion. Remember that acute diaphragmatic (inferior) MI is commonly due to right coronary artery occlusion, which also often causes various A-V junctional arrhythmias, including nonparoxysmal A-V JT.

The diagnosis of acute diaphragmatic MI can be made without any difficulty on the basis of abnormal Q waves in leads II, III, and aVF associated with ST segment elevation and T wave inversion. In addition, posterior myocardial ischemia is strongly considered because of tall T waves in leads V_{1-3}. Posterior ischemia or posterior MI is commonly associated with acute diaphragmatic MI and/or lateral MI.

By and large, nonparoxysmal A-V JT is a transient arrhythmia associated with acute diaphragmatic MI, and it is self-limited in most cases. Therefore no treatment is necessary.

A 67-year-old man who had suffered from a heart attack 2 years previously was examined in the ER for the evaluation of his new chest pain of several hours duration.

1. What is the ECG diagnosis?
2. What is the proper way to handle this patient?

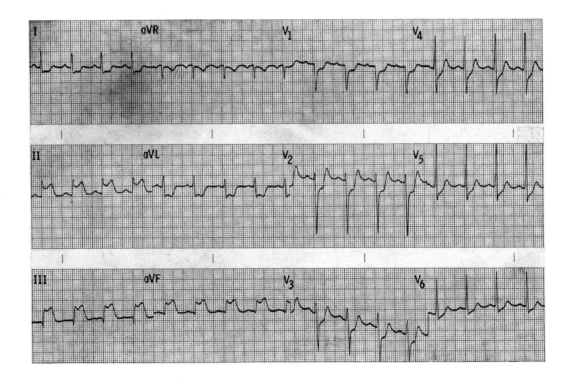

Diagnosis

The cardiac rhythm is sinus, with a rate of 100 beats per minute. There is evidence of diaphragmatic (inferior) MI, which he had suffered 2 years ago. His new ECG abnormality is marked ST segment elevation in leads II, III, and aVF associated with marked ST segment depression in V_{1-4} (lesser ST segment depression in leads V_{5-6}). This ECG finding represents acute diaphragmatic and posterior subepicardial injury.

Unless serial ECG tracings are obtained during close observation in the CCU, it will be impossible to determine whether these ST segment changes represent the early signs of superimposed acute MI or simply a coexisting subepicardial injury due to coronary artery spasm (see Case 2). Of course, serial serum enzyme studies further confirm or exclude the diagnosis of acute MI.

The patient was closely monitored and observed in the CCU for several days with conventional acute coronary care. He was found *not* to have a new acute MI at this time. He responded well to calcium channel blocker, and his chest pain as well as ST segment alterations subsided immediately.

CASE 7

This ECG tracing was obtained from a 78-year-old man with CAD. He had suffered from a heart attack 3 months previously, and his post-MI course was uneventful. He has been asymptomatic.

1. What is the ECG diagnosis?
2. Is an artificial pacemaker indicated?

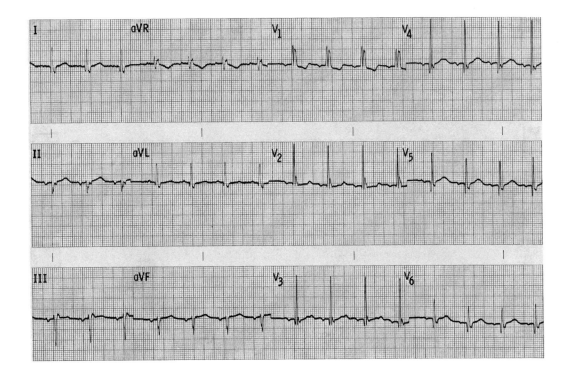

Diagnosis

Some inexperienced readers may erroneously consider that the cardiac rhythm is sinus simply because there are regularly occurring P waves followed by QRS complexes. However, more experienced readers should be able to recognize that all P waves are conducted in retrograde fashion (the P axis: -90 degrees).

The correct cardiac rhythm diagnosis is nonparoxysmal A-V JT with a rate of 87 beats per minute. An alternative rhythm diagnosis is coronary sinus rhythm.

Even inexperienced readers should be able to make the diagnosis of RBBB, but the coexisting posterolateral MI may not be recognized readily. The diagnosis of posterior MI is made on the basis of tall R wave (the first R wave among RR' in RBBB) in lead V_1, whereas abnormal Q waves in leads V_{4-6} are due to lateral MI. In addition, there is left anterior hemiblock (the QRS axis: -60 degrees). Thus a combination of RBBB and left anterior hemiblock represents BFB, which is a form of incomplete BBBB. Various ECG manifestations of BBBB are summarized as follows:

Diagnostic Criteria of BBBB (BFB and TFB)

1. RBBB with left anterior hemiblock.
2. RBBB with left posterior hemiblock.
3. Alternating left and right bundle branch block.
4. LBBB or RBBB with first-degree or second-degree A-V block.
5. LBBB or RBBB with prolonged H-V interval > 55 ms.
6. LBBB on one occasion and RBBB on another occasion.
7. Mobitz type II A-V block.
8. Any combination of the above findings.
9. Complete A-V block with VER (idioventricular).

Artificial pacing is not indicated for chronic BFB with or without MI.

CASE 8

A 72-year-man was admitted to the CCU because a heart attack was suspected. He has been relatively healthy, with only mild hypertension before this admission.

1. What is the ECG diagnosis?

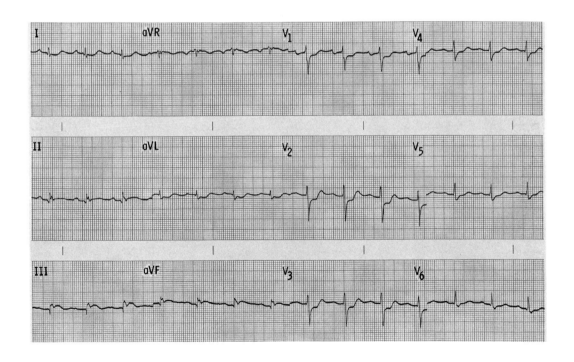

Diagnosis

The cardiac rhythm is sinus, with a rate of 82 beats per minute, and there is first degree A-V block (the PR interval: 0.22 second).

Most readers should be able to diagnose acute diaphragmatic (inferior) MI on the basis of abnormal Q waves in leads II, III, and aVF associated with ST segment elevation. In addition, posterior subepicardial injury is also present (ST segment depression in leads V_{1-3}). Posterolateral MI is a possibility because of relatively tall R waves in leads V_{1-3} along with poor progression of R waves in leads V_{4-6} with small Q waves in leads I and V_6.

Another ECG abnormality is low voltage of the QRS complexes, a common finding in patients with acute MI (see Case 4). Furthermore, the diagnosis of left atrial enlargement is made (note a broad and deep negative component of P wave in lead V_1). The QRS duration is slightly prolonged, and this finding is also common in patients with MI. This ECG abnormality is termed "diffuse" or "nonspecific intraventricular block."

CASE 9

A 68-year-old man was brought to the ER because of chest pain with acute onset associated with rapid heart action. He was *not* taking any medication.

1. What is the cardiac rhythm diagnosis?

2. What is the ECG diagnosis?
3. What is the treatment of choice for his arrhythmia?

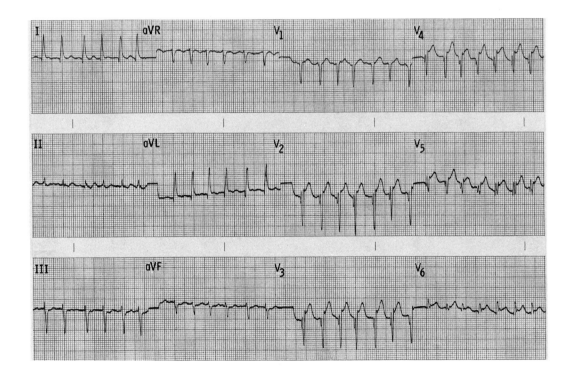

Diagnosis

The cardiac rhythm is AF, with rapid ventricular response (rate: 160–175 beats per minute). The characteristic features of AF is a grossly irregular ventricular cycle without any P waves. The atrial fibrillatory waves may be so small and ill-defined that the atrial activity appears to be absent in many cases of AF, especially in elderly people. Uncomplicated and untreated AF usually exhibits very rapid ventricular response (at least more than 120–140 beats per minute).

Acute extensive anterior MI is diagnosed without any difficulty on the basis of Q or QS waves in leads V_{1-6} associated with ST segment elevation.

The drug of choice for AF with rapid ventricular response is rapid digitalization, regardless of the clinical circumstance. The dosage of digitalization should be reduced considerably in patients with acute MI. When the clinical situation is extremely urgent, DC shock should be applied immediately.

CASE 10

This ECG tracing was obtained from a 58-year-old woman who has been treated for mild hypertension and intermittent chest pain for several months.

    1. What is the ECG diagnosis?

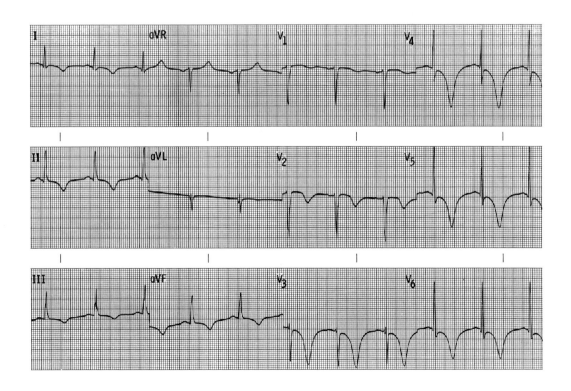

Diagnosis

The cardiac rhythm is sinus, with a rate of 62 beats per minute. The diagnosis of LVH can be entertained using the standard diagnostic criteria as follows:

Diagnostic Criteria of LVH

1. R wave in lead V_5 or $V_6 \geq 26$ mm.
2. R wave in lead V_5 or V_6 plus S wave in lead $V_1 \geq 35$ mm.
3. R wave in lead I ≥ 15 mm.
4. R wave in lead I plus S wave in lead III ≥ 25 mm.
5. R wave in lead aVL ≥ 13 mm or R wave in lead II, III, or aVF ≥ 20 mm.
6. Secondary T wave change (strain pattern) in leads V_{4-6} (only systolic overload).

Among these criteria the secondary T wave change (strain pattern) in leads V_{4-6} is the most important finding for definitive diagnosis of LVH. The reason for this is that many healthy young individuals and slender people will show very high left ventricular voltage without any abnormality of T waves.

Another ECG abnormality is inverted T waves involving many leads diffusely. This ECG finding is indicative of diffuse myocardial ischemia. The QT interval is significantly prolonged, and this ECG abnormality is not uncommon in patients with CAD.

Subendocardial infarction is considered when diffusely inverted T waves persist for many days, especially associated with considerable chest pain.

CASE 11

A heart attack was suspected in a 55-year-old obese woman. She was *not* taking any medication.

  1. What is the ECG diagnosis?

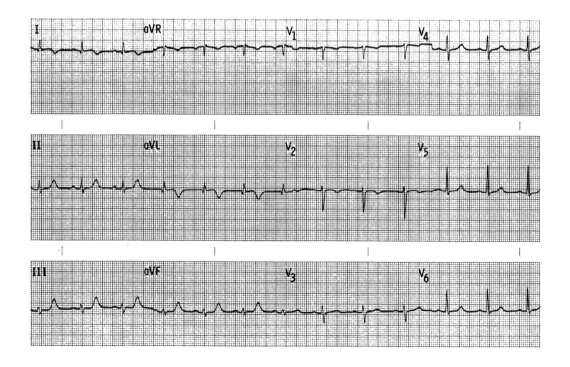

Diagnosis

The cardiac rhythm is sinus, with a rate of 74 beats per minute. The abnormal findings are shown only in leads I and aVL. These two leads reveal abnormal Q waves with ST segment elevation and T wave inversion diagnostic of acute, high, lateral MI. Thus this is a good example of a very localized MI involving only high lateral wall of the left ventricle.

The T waves are slightly inverted in leads V_{1-2}, suggestive of anteroseptal myocardial ischemia. In addition, there is low voltage of the QRS complexes (see Case 4).

CASE 12

This ECG tracing was taken on a 56-year-old man with a previous history of heart attack. The tracing was performed a few hours following CABS.

   1. What is the ECG diagnosis?

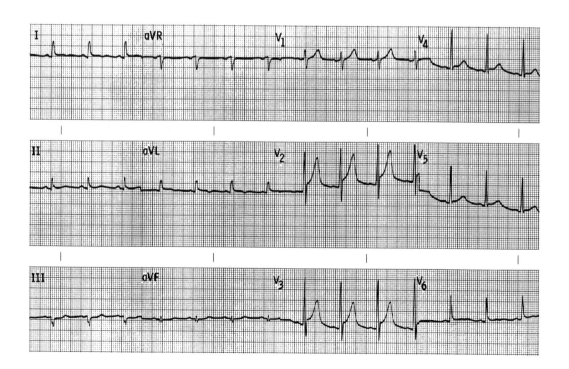

Diagnosis

The cardiac rhythm is sinus, with a rate of 86 beats per minute. The ST segment is elevated diffusely in many leads as a result of CABS-induced acute pericarditis (*see* Case 3).

Another ECG abnormality is posterior MI, which is manifested by a relatively tall R wave in lead V_1 with a tall T wave. Remember that posterior MI does *not* produce an abnormal Q wave because there is no ECG lead that directly records the elec-

tric event occurring in the posterior wall of the left ventricle. Thus only indirect evidence of posterior MI is registered in lead V_1 as a tall or relatively tall R wave (reciprocal change). In reality a tall or relatively tall R wave in lead V_1 represents a pathologic Q wave if the posterior ECG lead is used. Posterior MI often coexists with diaphragmatic and/or lateral MI (*see* Cases 13, 14, 18, 19, 25, 26, 31, 32, 39, and 43).

A 47-year-old man was admitted to the CCU because MI was diagnosed in the ER. His risk factors for CAD include a strong family history of CAD, cigarette smoking, and obesity. He was *not* taking any drug before this admission.

1. What is the ECG diagnosis?
2. What is the proper way to handle this patient?

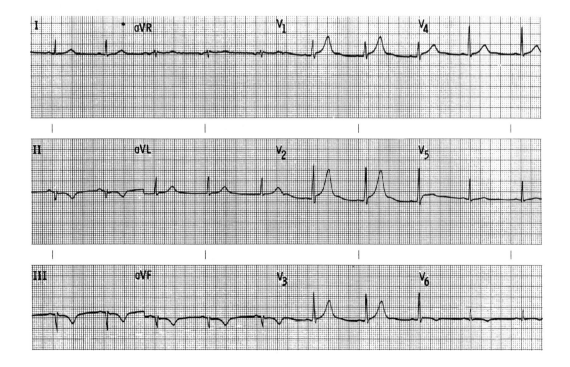

Diagnosis

The cardiac rhythm is sinus, with a rate of 61 beats per minute. Abnormal ECG findings in this tracing include pathologic Q waves with T wave inversion in leads II, III, aVF, and V_6 associated with tall R waves in leads V_{1-3} with tall T waves. Thus the diagnosis of diaphragmatic posterolateral MI can be made without much difficulty. It should be noted again that there will be no Q wave in posterior MI because there is no ECG lead that directly records any electric event occurring in the posterior wall (*see* Case 12).

The patient underwent coronary arteriography to determine the exact degree and location of coronary artery lesion(s) for possible PTCA or CABS as indicated.

This ECG tracing was obtained from a 55-year-old man with CAD.

1. What is the ECG diagnosis?
2. Is an artificial pacemaker indicated?

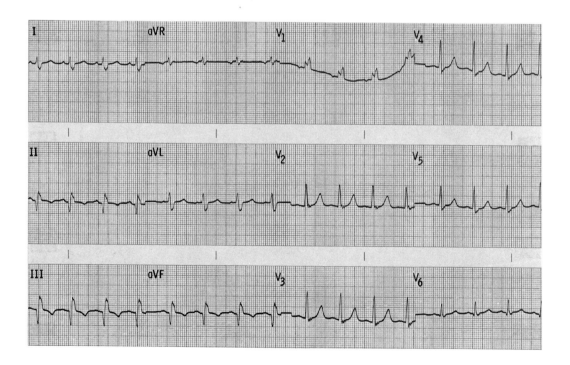

Diagnosis

The cardiac rhythm is sinus, with a rate of 90 beats per minute. The diagnosis of diaphragmatic posterolateral MI can be entertained by most experienced readers, but inexperienced readers may feel some difficulty in recognizing posterior MI in the presence of RBBB. It should be emphasized that the first R wave among RR' in lead V_1 is wider and taller than a pure RBBB, as a result of posterior MI. Actually there is complete loss of posterior force (all components of the QRS complex in lead V_1 are upright without any negative QRS component below the baseline PR and ST segment).

Artificial pacing is *not* indicated for RBBB with acute or old MI (regardless of the location of MI).

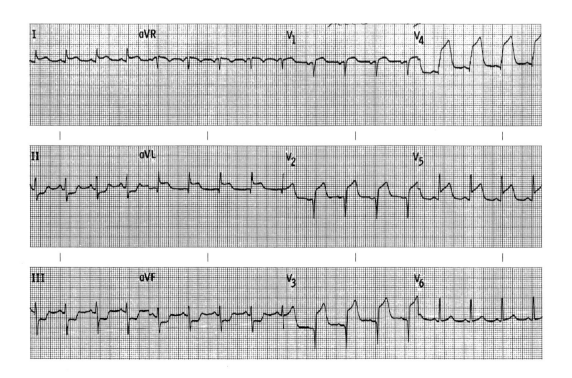

CASE 15

A 74-year-old man was admitted to the CCU because acute MI was diagnosed.

1. What is the ECG diagnosis?

Diagnosis

The cardiac rhythm is sinus, with a rate of 96 beats per minute. The diagnosis of acute anteroseptal MI can be made without much difficulty on the basis of Q or QS waves in leads V_{1-4} associated with marked ST segment elevation in leads I, aVL, and V_{1-5}.

The ST segment depression in leads II, III, and aVF probably represents reciprocal change, but coexisting diaphragmatic (inferior) subendocardial injury is also considered. The ST segment elevation in leads I and aVL represents high lateral subepicardial injury.

This ECG tracing was obtained from a 75-year-old man with severe chest pain of a few hours duration.

    1. What is the ECG diagnosis?

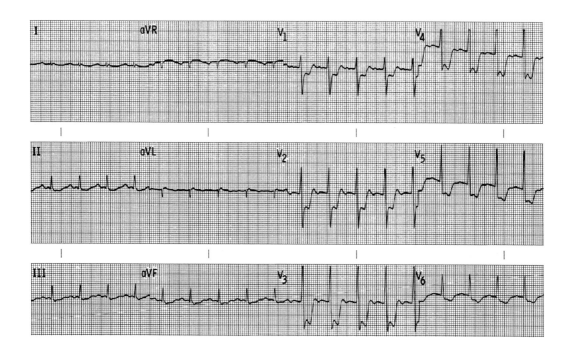

Diagnosis

The cardiac rhythm is sinus tachycardia, with a rate of 106 beats per minute. The striking ECG abnormality in this tracing is marked ST segment depression in leads V_{1-6}. This ECG finding may represent either posterior subepicardial injury or anterior subendocardial injury. It is rather difficult to differentiate these two processes if only one ECG tracing is available. However, most likely posterior subepicardial injury is the correct diagnosis judging from the fact that the ST segment depression is most pronounced in leads V_{2-4}.

The patient expired soon after admission to the CCU. There is low voltage of the QRS complexes (*see* Case 4). Relatively tall R wave in lead V_1 is suggestive of posterior MI (*see* Case 12).

CASE 17

A 57-year-old man who has a history of a heart attack 2 years previously was readmitted to the CCU because another heart attack was suspected.

1. What is the ECG diagnosis?

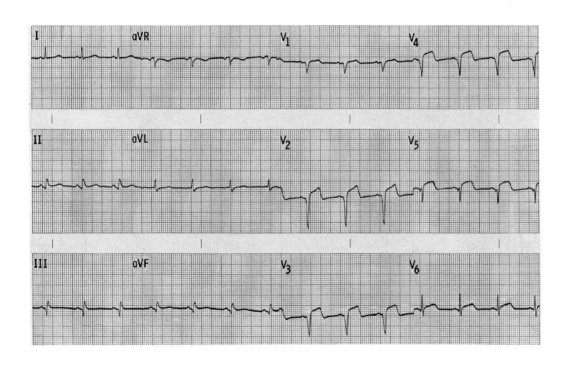

Diagnosis

The cardiac rhythm is sinus, with a rate of 78 beats per minute. Acute extensive (massive) anterior MI is obvious, which is manifested by QS waves in leads V_{1-5} associated with marked ST segment elevation and T wave inversion.

In addition, there is old diaphragmatic (inferior) MI, which is manifested by pathologic Q waves in leads III and aVF and a small Q wave in lead II. Another ECG abnormality is low voltage of the QRS complexes (*see* Case 4).

CASE 18

A 50-year-old obese woman with known CAD was examined in the ER because of recurrent chest pain.

1. What is the ECG diagnosis?

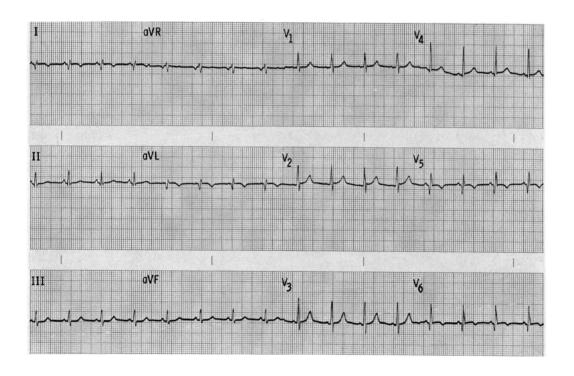

Diagnosis

The cardiac rhythm is sinus, with a rate of 90 beats per minute. The diagnosis of posterior MI can be entertained on the basis of tall R waves in leads V_{1-3} with upright T waves (see Case 12). In addition, lateral (including high lateral) MI is diagnosed (see Case 11) on the basis of Q waves in leads I, aVL, and V_{5-6} associated with ST segment elevation and T wave inversion.

Thus the diagnosis of posterolateral MI is made.

Her MI is considered to be approximately two to three days old judging from a clinical history and the ECG findings.

Another ECG finding is low voltage of the QRS complexes (see Case 4)—very common in patients with recent MI.

A 44-year-old man with multiple risk factors for CAD was seen at the cardiac clinic during a periodic follow-up examination. He was found to be relatively asymptomatic.

1. What is the ECG diagnosis?

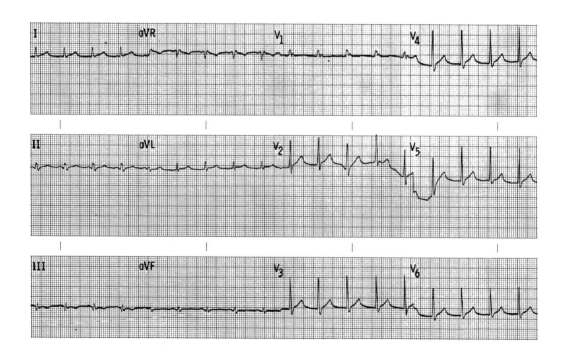

Diagnosis

The cardiac rhythm is sinus tachycardia, with a rate of 102 beats per minute. The diagnosis of incomplete RBBB can be made even by most inexperienced readers without much difficulty. However, coexisting posterior MI may *not* be recognized readily by some readers. Posterior MI is strongly considered because the initial R wave (among RR') in lead V_1 is broad and tall. In addition, diaphragmatic MI is most likely present. Thus this patient had suffered from diaphragmatic and posterior MI.

Furthermore, some experienced readers may raise a possibility of right ventricular MI because the second R wave (among RR') in lead V_1 is very small, and the depth of the S waves in leads V_{4-6} is minimum. Remember that the second R wave in lead V_1 in RBBB and S waves in leads V_{4-6} are due to delayed right ventricular activation. When right ventricular MI occurs, obviously the amplitude of these waves will be diminished because of the right ventricular dysfunction. Right ventricular MI frequently coexists with diaphragmatic, posterior, and/or lateral MI.

Another ECG abnormality is low voltage of the QRS complexes (*see* Case 4).

The PR interval is shorter than usual, but this finding is a normal variant. Short PR interval is *not* uncommon in healthy young adults and children as well as in any individual during stressful situations.

This ECG tracing was obtained from a 68-year-old man who had suffered from a heart attack 1 year earlier. He has been doing relatively well with maintenance oral digoxin therapy (0.25 mg).

1. What is the cardiac rhythm diagnosis?
2. What is the ECG diagnosis?

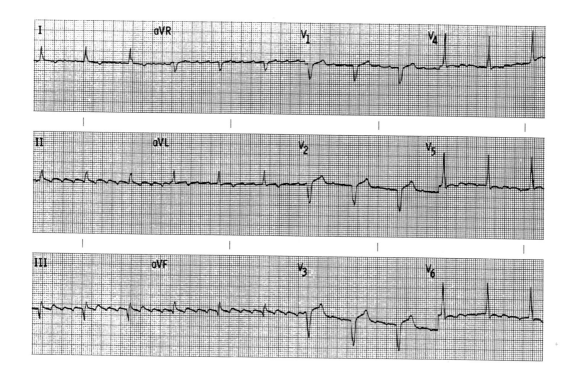

Diagnosis

The underlying rhythm is atrial flutter (atrial rate: 268 beats per minute) with 4:1 A-V block (ventricular rate: 67 beats per minute).

There are evidences of old diaphragmatic MI (Q waves in leads II, III, and aVF) and anteroseptal MI (QS waves in leads V_{1-3}). The QRS interval is slightly wider than usual—nonspecific (diffuse) intraventricular block.

CASE 21

A 68-year-old man was examined in a cardiologist's office for the evaluation of his recurrent chest pain of several weeks duration. He was not taking any cardiac drug.

1. What is the ECG diagnosis?
2. What is the proper way to handle this patient?

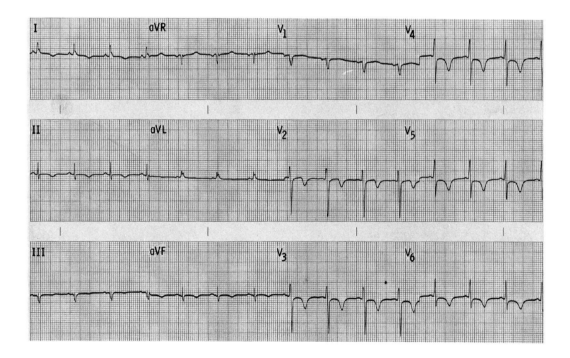

Diagnosis

The cardiac rhythm is sinus, with a rate of 82 beats per minute. Inverted T waves that involve inferior as well as entire precordial leads are obvious. Thus diffuse myocardial ischemia is diagnosed (*see* Cases 1 and 10).

He was admitted to the CCU for in-depth evaluation of his chest pain and because of his markedly abnormal ECG. When acute MI was excluded, he underwent coronary arteriography to determine his coronary artery lesion(s) for possible PTCA or CABS as indicated.

This ECG tracing was taken several hours following CABS on a 51-year-old man with CAD.

1. What is the ECG diagnosis?

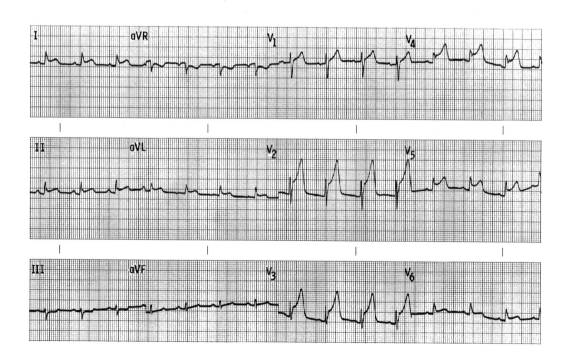

Diagnosis

The cardiac rhythm is sinus, with a rate of 84 beats per minute. The diagnosis of posterolateral MI is strongly considered on the basis of a relatively tall R wave in lead V_1 with upright T wave and poor progression of R waves in leads V_{4-6} (see Cases 8 and 18).

The ST segment is elevated in many leads, indicative of acute pericarditis as a result of CABS (a form of postcardiotomy syndrome, see Cases 3 and 12).

CASE 23

A 56-year-old man with known CAD came to the cardiac clinic for a periodic follow-up examination. He had been doing well without any significant cardiac symptom.

   1. What is the ECG diagnosis?

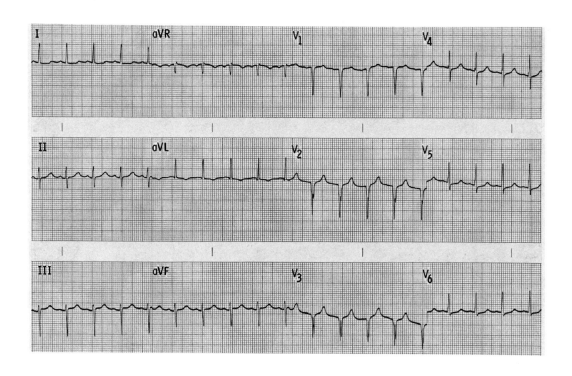

Diagnosis

The cardiac rhythm is sinus tachycardia, with a rate of 110 beats per minute.

The diagnosis of old anteroseptal MI can be made without much difficulty on the basis of QS waves in leads V_{1-3}. In addition, there is left axis deviation of the QRS complexes (the QRS axis: -25 degrees). He had suffered from a heart attack 3 years previously, and his post-MI recovery was uneventful.

A 70-year-old man was admitted to the CCU because the diagnosis of recent heart attack was established in the ER.

1. What is the ECG diagnosis?

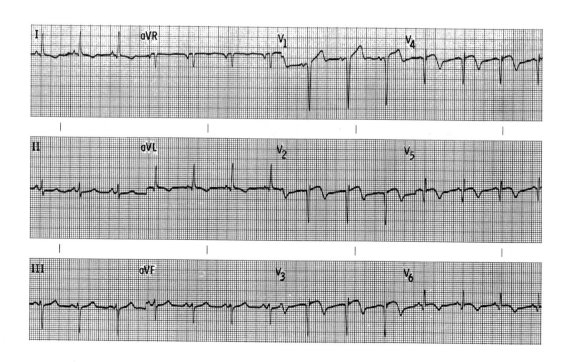

Diagnosis

The cardiac rhythm is sinus, with a rate of 78 beats per minute.

It should be noted that QS waves or pathologic Q waves are present in the entire precordial leads associated with ST segment elevation and T wave inversion. Thus the diagnosis of acute extensive anterior MI is entertained (*see* Case 4).

In addition, LVH is strongly considered (*see* Case 10).

This ECG tracing was recorded from a 59-year-old man with CAD.

1. What is the ECG diagnosis?

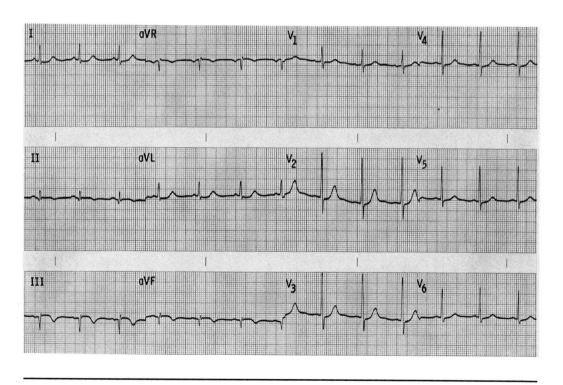

Diagnosis

The cardiac rhythm is sinus, with a rate of 76 beats per minute.

The diagnosis of diaphragmatic MI can be made readily on the basis of pathologic Q waves in leads II, III, and aVF associated with ST segment elevation and T wave inversion. In addition, there is evidence of posterior MI on the basis of a tall R wave in lead V_1 with upright T wave. Thus the diagnosis of diaphragmatic and posterior MI is fully established (*see* Case 19).

A 55-year-old man with previous history of a heart attack was examined in a cardiologist's office during a routine medical checkup.

    1. What is the ECG diagnosis?

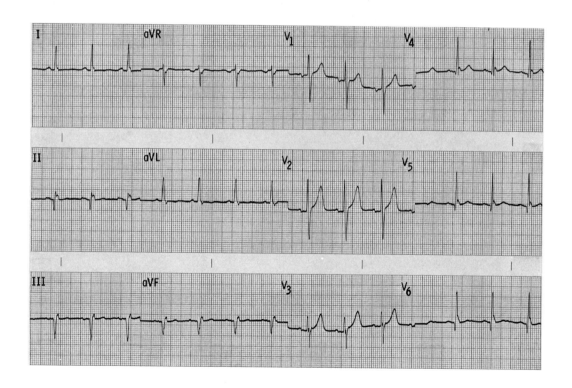

Diagnosis

The cardiac rhythm is sinus, with a rate of 84 beats per minute.

The diagnosis of diaphragmatic-lateral MI can be made readily even by most inexperienced readers on the basis of pathologic Q waves in leads II, III, aVF, and V_{5-6}. However, coexisting posterior MI may *not* be diagnosed by some readers. The relatively tall R wave in lead V_1 with upright T wave is diagnostic of posterior MI. Thus this patient had suffered from diaphragmatic posterolateral MI (*see* Case 13).

In addition, LAH is considered.

CASE 27

A 47-year-old man with a history of cigarette smoking for many years was admitted to the CCU because a heart attack was suspected.

1. What is the ECG diagnosis?
2. Is an artificial pacemaker indicated?

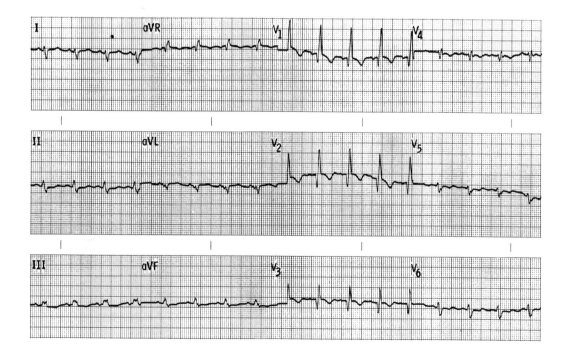

Diagnosis

The cardiac rhythm is sinus, with a rate of 100 beats per minute.

The diagnosis of BFB consisting of RBBB and left posterior hemiblock (the QRS axis: +130 degrees) can be made by most experienced readers. However, a co-existing anteroseptal MI in the presence of RBBB or BFB is often missed by some readers. In fact, many patients develop RBBB or BFB as a result of acute anteroseptal or anterior MI, as seen in this case.

The diagnostic criteria of BBBB are summarized in Case 7. Remember that BFB is a form of incomplete BBBB.

The diagnostic criteria of hemiblocks are summarized as follows:

Diagnostic Criteria of Left Anterior Hemiblock

1. Marked left axis deviation (−45 to −90 degrees) of QRS complexes.
2. Small Q wave in lead I and small R wave in lead III.
3. Little or no prolongation of QRS interval.

4. No evidence of other factors responsible for left axis deviation (true or pseudo).

Diagnostic Criteria of Left Posterior Hemiblock

1. Marked right axis deviation (+105 to +180 degrees) of QRS complexes.
2. Small R wave in lead I and small Q wave in lead III.
3. Little or no prolongation of QRS interval.
4. No evidence of other factors responsible for right axis deviation (true or pseudo).

The prophylactic artificial pacing is recommended for BFB with acute onset as a result of recent anteroseptal or anterior MI because these patients may develop more advanced forms of BBBB in the near future.

CASE 28

This ECG tracing was recorded from a 65-year-old man in the CCU.

1. What is the ECG diagnosis?
2. Is an artificial pacemaker indicated?

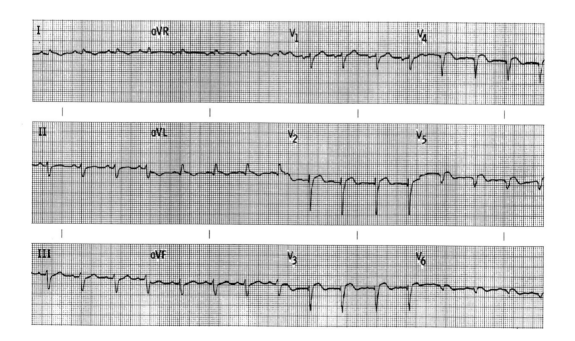

Diagnosis

The cardiac rhythm is sinus, with a rate of 92 beats per minute.

The diagnosis of extensive anterior MI (except for the ventricular septum) can be diagnosed without much difficulty even by inexperienced readers on the basis of QS waves or Q waves in leads V_{2-6}, I, and aVL associated with ST segment elevation and T wave inversion.

In addition, left anterior hemiblock is diagnosed using the conventional criteria (*see* Case 27). The QRS axis is calculated to be -65 degrees.

The prophylactic artificial pacing is *not* indicated for hemiblocks (acute or chronic) associated with recent MI.

CASE 29

This ECG tracing was obtained from a 43-year-old man with multiple risk factors for CAD (cigarette smoking, family history of CAD, obesity, and hypertension).

1. What is the ECG diagnosis?

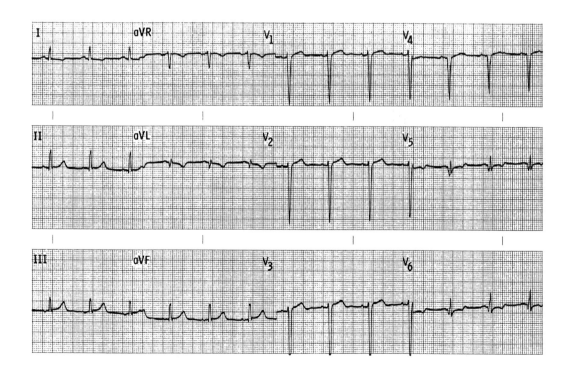

Diagnosis

The cardiac rhythm is sinus, with a rate of 75 beats per minute.

The diagnosis of anterolateral MI is established on the basis of Q or QS waves (or markedly reduced amplitude of R waves) in leads V_{4-6} with biphasic to inverted T waves in leads V_{5-6}. Anterolateral MI is often called simply "lateral MI." Thus lateral MI means anterolateral MI.

In addition, high lateral wall involvement is strongly considered on the basis of Q wave with inverted T wave in lead aVL (see Case 11).

Needless to say, this patient should be fully instructed to eliminate or control all risk factors to prevent a second or third heart attack. In particular, he must stop smoking instantly because cigarette smoking is found to be the strongest risk factor for CAD in young to middle-aged men according to a variety of epidemiologic studies.

CASE 30

A 71-year-old man was brought to the ER because he almost collapsed, and this episode was associated with severe chest pain and dyspnea of one hour duration.

1. What is the ECG diagnosis?
2. What is the proper way to handle this patient?

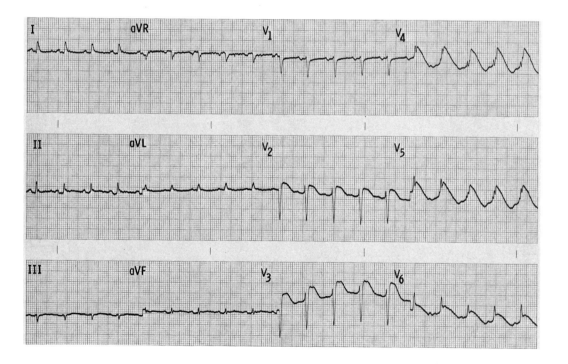

Diagnosis

The cardiac rhythm is sinus tachycardia, with a rate of 115 beats per minute.

The ST segment is markedly elevated in almost entire precordial leads so that it is difficult to separate the QRS complex, ST segment, and T wave in some ECG leads. The ST segment elevation in these chest leads represents diffuse anterior subepicardial injury, and there is poor progression of R waves in leads V_{3-6}. Thus these ECG findings are diagnostic of acute anterior MI, primarily involving the lateral wall of the left ventricle.

Of course the patient was immediately hospitalized in the CCU for routine acute coronary care. Since the MI is in its very early stage, this patient is an excellent candidate for intracoronary (or, less commonly, intravenous [IV]) streptokinase therapy. When the streptokinase therapy is ineffective, PTCA or CABS should be considered depending upon the clinical circumstance.

There is low voltage of the QRS complexes (*see* Case 4).

CASE 31

This ECG tracing was taken on a 70-year-old man with a previous history of a heart attack 6 months earlier.

1. What is the ECG diagnosis?

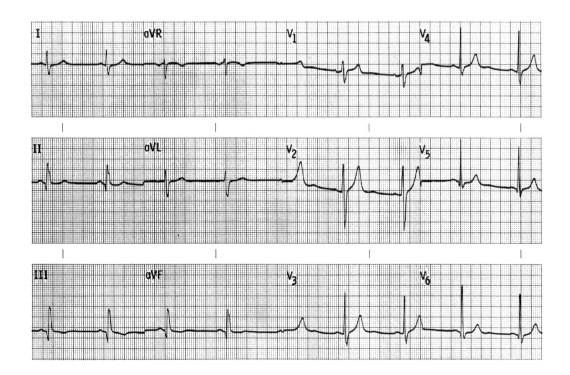

Diagnosis

The cardiac rhythm is sinus bradycardia, with a rate of 52 beats per minute.

Diaphragmatic (inferior) MI is diagnosed on the basis of pathologic Q waves in leads II, III, and aVF. In addition, the diagnosis of posterior MI is entertained on the basis of a relatively tall R wave in lead V_1 with upright T wave. Thus this ECG demonstrates diaphragmatic-posterior MI (see Case 19). It has been shown that diaphragmatic MI often coexists with posterior and/or lateral MI (see Cases 13, 14, 26, and 32).

CASE 32

A 51-year-old man with known CAD was
evaluated at the cardiac clinic for further
management of his cardiac problem.

1. What is the ECG diagnosis?

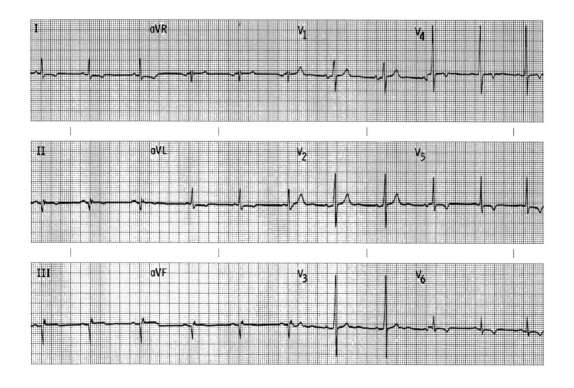

Diagnosis

The cardiac rhythm is sinus bradycardia, with a rate of 58 beats per minute.

The diagnosis of diaphragmatic-posterolateral MI can be established using the conventional diagnostic criteria (*see* Case 13). Namely, pathologic Q waves in leads II, III, and aVF are due to diaphragmatic MI, whereas markedly reduced amplitude of R wave in lead V_6 with Q wave represents lateral MI. Posterior MI is diagnosed on the basis of a relatively tall R wave in lead V_1 with upright T wave. As repeatedly emphasized, diaphragmatic-posterolateral MI is a common coexisting finding (*see* Cases 13, 14, and 26).

LAH is also considered.

This ECG tracing was discussed during a weekly ECG conference because of somewhat unusual abnormalities. The patient is a 55-year-old woman who was admitted to the CCU because of recurrent chest pain of a few weeks duration.

1. What is the ECG diagnosis?

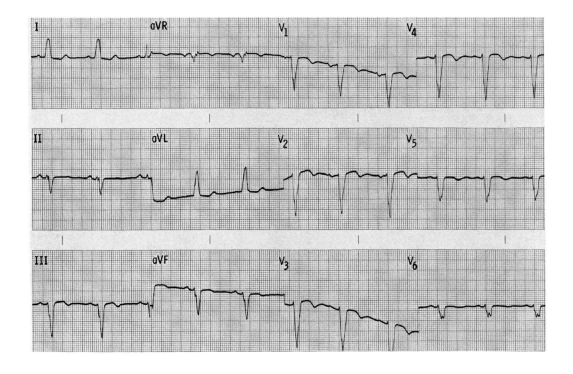

Diagnosis

The cardiac rhythm is sinus, with a rate of 62 beats per minute.

The diagnosis of LBBB can be made even by most inexperienced readers using conventional diagnostic criteria as follows:

Diagnostic Criteria of LBBB

1. QRS interval ≥ 0.12 second.
2. Absence of septal Q waves in leads I, aVL, and V_{4-6}.
3. RSR', "M" pattern, or broad R waves in leads I, aVL, and V_{4-6}.
4. Broad QS or RS waves in leads V_{1-3}.
5. Secondary, ST,T wave changes in leads I, aVL, and V_{4-6}.

However, the unusual feature of this ECG tracing is the T wave abnormality, namely, the primary T wave change replaced the secondary T wave change. Note that the T waves are inverted in leads III, aVF, and V_{1-6}, indicative of diffuse myocardial ischemia. In other words, diffuse myocardial ischemia coexists with LBBB. A pure LBBB is manifested by inverted or biphasic T waves in leads I, aVL, and V_{4-6}, with upright T waves in the remaining leads (see Case 66).

When the primary T wave change (ischemic change) occurs in the presence of LBBB, acute MI should be considered until proven otherwise.

In addition, the diagnosis of LAH is entertained. Most patients with LBBB show clinical and x-ray evidence of LVH, and often left atrial enlargement coexists.

The diagnostic criteria of left atrial hypertrophy are summarized as below:

Diagnostic Criteria of LAH

1. Wide (3 mm or more) and notched P waves in leads I, II, and aVL (less commonly in other limb leads).
2. Negative (inverted) component of P waves in leads $V_{1,2}$ with depth and width of 1 mm or more.
3. Coarse AF ("f" waves in lead V_1 or V_2, 1 mm or more in amplitude).

CASE 34

A 77-year-old man was admitted to the CCU via the ER because a heart attack was suspected.

1. What is the ECG diagnosis?
2. Is an artificial pacemaker indicated?

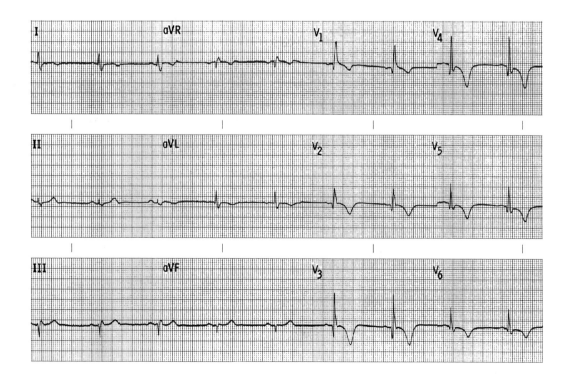

Diagnosis

This cardiac rhythm is sinus bradycardia, with a rate of 52 beats per minute.

The diagnosis of RBBB can be established without any difficulty using the conventional diagnostic criteria as follows:

Diagnostic Criteria of RBBB

1. QRS interval $\geq$ 0.12 second.
2. RSR' or "M" pattern of QRS in leads V_{1-3}.
3. Deep and slurred S waves in leads I, aVL, and V_{4-6}.
4. Secondary ST, T wave change in leads V_{1-3}.

The coexisting ECG abnormality is recent, extensive, anterior MI, which is manifested by pathologic Q waves in leads V_{1-6} associated with T wave inversion and ST segment elevation in leads V_{1-3} (*see* Case 4).

It should be remembered that a pure RBBB reveals RR' of QRS complexes in leads V_{1-3} with biphasic to inverted T waves (often ST segment depression also), and the remaining leads demonstrate upright T waves. No pathologic Q waves are shown in a pure RBBB (*see* Case 65).

The prophylactic pacing is *not* recommended for RBBB even if it is produced by acute anterior MI.

CASE 35

A 76-year-old man with long-standing hypertension and known CAD was evaluated at the cardiac clinic as a periodic medical checkup.

    1. What is the ECG diagnosis?

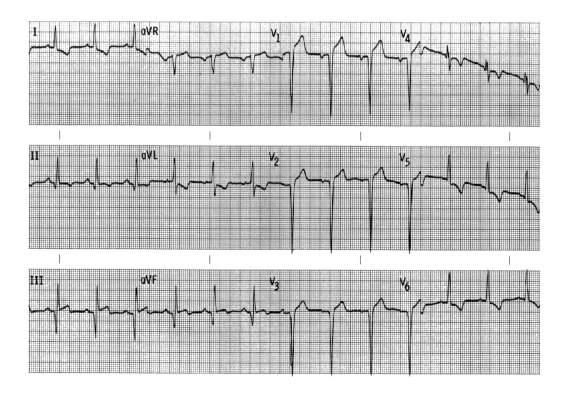

Diagnosis

The cardiac rhythm is sinus, with a rate of 77 beats per minute.

There are several ECG abnormalities. The first ECG abnormality is diaphragmatic (inferior) MI, which is manifested by pathologic Q waves in leads II, III, and aVF associated with T wave inversion and slight ST segment elevation.

The second abnormality is anteroseptal MI, which is manifested by QS waves in leads V_{1-3}.

The third ECG finding is LVH. The diagnostic criteria of LVH have been described previously (see Case 10). Needless to say, the commonest cause of LVH is systemic hypertension, and LAH (the fourth ECG abnormality) often coexists (see diagnostic criteria of LAH, Case 33).

When the ST segment elevation persists more than a week following an acute MI or the ST segment elevation reappears, ventricular aneurysm should be considered (see Case 41). However, not uncommonly ST segment elevation may persist for many weeks, months, or even indefinitely following MI without any reason. Likewise the T wave inversion may last for long periods of time after MI without any particular reason.

CASE 36

A 61-year-old man was seen in the ER because he developed chest pain suddenly.

1. What is the ECG diagnosis?

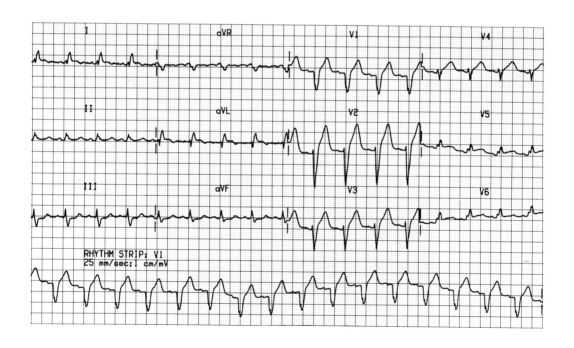

Diagnosis

The cardiac rhythm is sinus, with a rate of 100 beats per minute.

The diagnosis of LBBB can be made without much difficulty using the conventional diagnostic criteria (*see* Case 33). However, the ST segment elevation with upright T waves in leads I, aVL, and V_{5-6} is a very unusual feature of LBBB, namely, anterolateral subepicardial injury with ischemia is superimposed in the presence of LBBB. Thus coronary artery spasm or acute MI involving lateral wall should be strongly considered.

It should be noted that a pure form of LBBB reveals biphasic or slightly inverted T waves in leads I, aVL, and V_{4-6} associated with ST segment depression (or isolectric ST segment, *see* Case 66).

This patient should be monitored in the CCU for acute coronary care until the final diagnosis (acute MI versus coronary artery spasm) is fully established so that proper definitive treatment can be provided.

CASE 37

This ECG tracing was taken on a 77-year-old woman with known CAD while she was experiencing chest pain.

1. What is the ECG diagnosis?

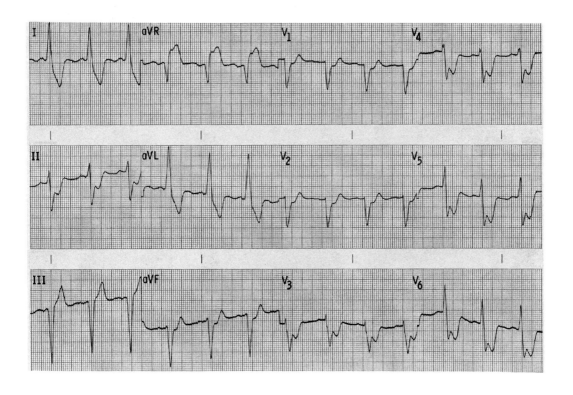

Diagnosis

The cardiac rhythm is sinus, with a rate of 76 beats per minute.

Most readers should be able to diagnose LBBB using the conventional diagnostic criteria (see Case 33). However, some inexperienced readers may fail to recognize more-than-usual ST segment depression in many leads, namely the ST segment is markedly depressed in leads II and V_{3-6}, indicative of inferolateral subendocardial injury.

When marked ST segment depression (horizontal to downsloping) persists more than several days, subendocardial MI should strongly be considered.

CASE 38

A 71-year-old man was examined in his physician's office during a periodic medical checkup. This patient had suffered from a heart attack several years ago, but his post-MI recovery was uneventful.

1. What is the ECG diagnosis?

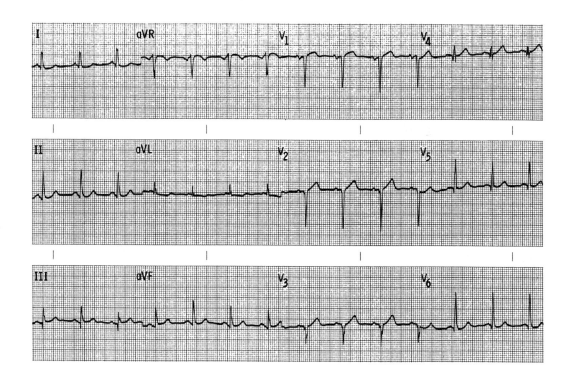

Diagnosis

The cardiac rhythm is sinus, with a rate of 82 beats per minute.

In the precordial leads there is almost loss of R waves in leads V_{1-3} as a result of old anteroseptal MI. The T waves are upright in these chest leads, and there is no ST segment elevation.

In addition, old diaphragmatic (inferior) MI is a possibility in view of a relatively large Q wave in lead III with a small Q wave in lead aVF.

CASE 39

A 51-year-old man was admitted to the CCU via the ER because of severe chest pain of a few hours duration.

1. What is the ECG diagnosis?
2. What is the proper way of handling this patient?

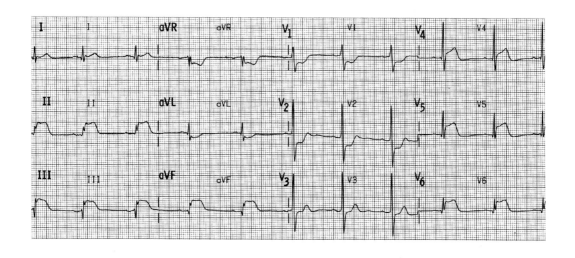

Diagnosis

The cardiac rhythm is sinus, with a rate of 60 beats per minute.

The ST segment is markedly elevated in leads II, III, aVF, and V_{4-6}, indicative of acute diaphragmatic-lateral subepicardial injury. There is markedly reduced amplitude of R waves with or without Q waves in leads II, III, aVF, and V_{5-6}. Thus the diagnosis of acute diaphragmatic-lateral MI is established.

Another ECG abnormality is a relatively tall R wave in lead V_1 with marked ST segment depression in leads V_{1-2} diagnostic of acute posterior MI.

When the above-mentioned ECG abnormalities are interpreted together, the diagnosis of acute diaphragmatic-posterolateral MI is fully made (see Case 13). It has been shown that MI often involves simultaneously diaphragmatic wall, posterior wall as well as lateral wall of the left ventricle (see Cases 13, 14, 26, and 32).

Since his MI occurred only a few hours ago, intracoronary streptokinase therapy should be considered first. If this therapeutic approach fails, PTCA or CABS should be the next step, depending upon the clinical circumstance.

CASE 40

This ECG tracing was discussed during a weekly ECG conference. A 64-year-old man was admitted to the CCU because of a recent heart attack.

1. What is the ECG diagnosis?
2. Is an artificial pacemaker indicated?

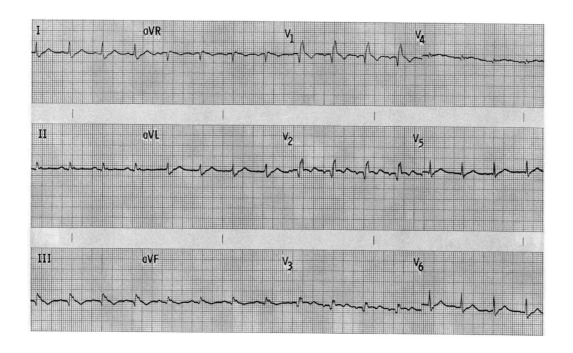

Diagnosis

The cardiac rhythm is sinus, with a rate of 92 beats per minute.

The diagnosis of RBBB can be made by most readers using the conventional diagnostic criteria (*see* Case 34). However, coexisting ECG abnormality may not be recognized by some inexperienced readers.

There are pathologic Q waves in leads II, III, and aVF, with ST segment elevation and T wave inversion in leads III and aVF. These ECG findings are diagnostic of recent diaphragmatic MI.

Another ECG abnormality is pathologic Q waves in leads V_{1-4}, with ST segment elevation and inverted T waves in leads V_{1-3}, indicative of recent anteroseptal MI.

The prophylactic pacing is not indicated for RBBB associated with recent MI.

CASE 41

A 50-year-old man with a history of a heart attack 2 months previously was referred to the cardiac clinic because of persisting ST segment elevation in many leads associated with CHF. He has been taking a maintenance digoxin 0.25 mg daily.

1. What is the ECG diagnosis?
2. What is the proper way of handling this patient?

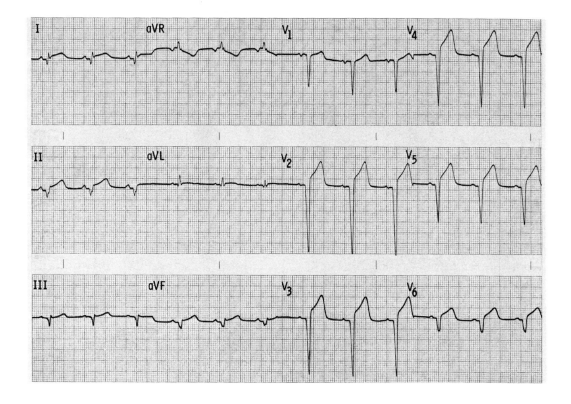

Diagnosis

The cardiac rhythm is sinus, with a rate of 72 beats per minute.

It is obvious to diagnose diaphragmatic and extensive anterior MI in view of Q waves or QS waves in leads II, III, aVF, and V_{1-6}.

Ventricular aneurysm should be strongly considered when the ST segment elevation persists more than 1 week following an acute MI.

A cardiac surgeon was consulted immediately for possible ventricular aneurysmectomy.

There is low voltage of the QRS complexes (see Case 4).

CASE 42

This ECG tracing was obtained from a 59-year-old woman with a temporary pacemaker.

1. What is the ECG diagnosis?
2. What is the mode of artificial pacing?

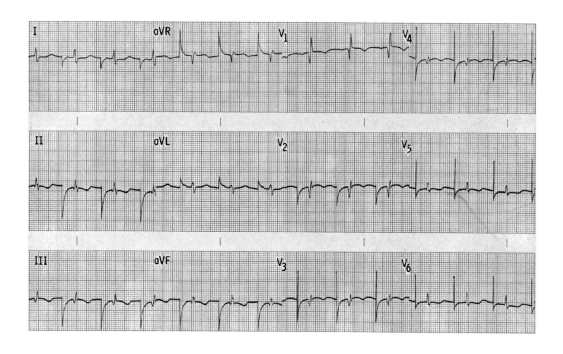

Diagnosis

The cardiac rhythm is atrial or coronary sinus pacemaker, with a rate of 74 beats per minute. Note that each pacemaker spike initiates the P wave in the atrial or coronary sinus pacemaker rhythm, but the P waves (usually retrograde P waves) are often *not* clearly visible.

The diagnosis of diaphragmatic and extensive anterior MI is established on the basis of Q waves in II, III, aVF, and V_{1-6} associated with T wave inversion and ST segment elevation.

Another ECG abnormality is incomplete RBBB (*see* Case 34).

CASE 43

This ECG tracing, which belongs to a 67-year-old man with CAD, was presented to the Cardiology Grand Round because of several interesting features.

1. What is the ECG diagnosis?

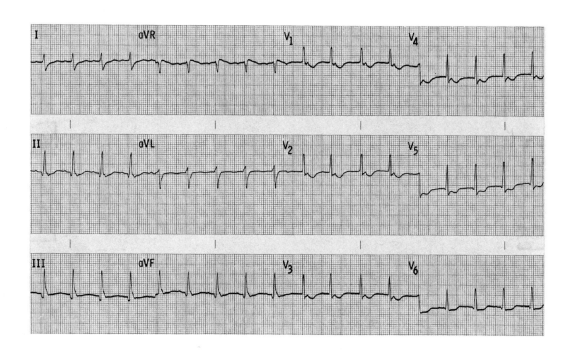

Diagnosis

The cardiac rhythm is sinus tachycardia, with a rate of 101 beats per minute.

The diagnosis of diaphragmatic MI is established on the basis of Q waves in leads II, III, and aVF. In addition, the diagnosis of posterior MI is a coexisting abnormality on the basis of tall R waves in leads V_{1-3}. Furthermore, lateral MI is also considered because the amplitude of R wave is diminished with a small Q wave in lead V_6.

Some experienced readers may raise another possible diagnosis. Namely, right ventricular MI is considered because the amplitude of second R waves of RR' in RBBB are smaller than expected in leads V_{1-3}, with small S waves in leads V_{4-6} (see Case 19).

Of course the diagnosis of RBBB is obvious, but the configuration of the QRS complexes is altered because of the coexisting posterior MI and possible right ventricular MI. It has been shown that right ventricular MI usually coexists with diaphragmatic MI.

CHAPTER TWO

CHAMBER ENLARGEMENT (HYPERTROPHY)

This ECG tracing was obtained from a 61-year-old woman with mitral stenosis due to RHD. She has been relatively asymptomatic except for some exercise intolerance.

1. What is the ECG diagnosis?

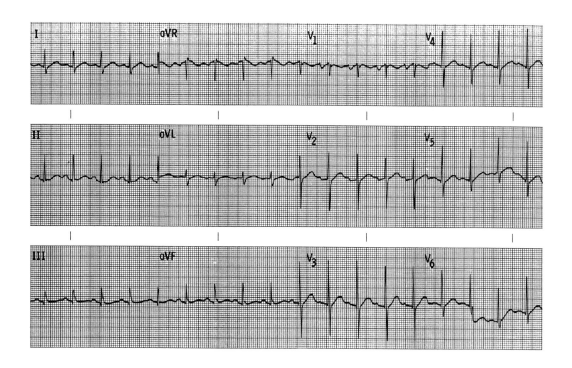

Diagnosis

The cardiac rhythm is sinus tachycardia, with a rate of 105 beats per minute.

The only abnormality in this ECG tracing is left atrial enlargement. Note that the P waves are broad in many limb leads, and that they are notched. In addition, the negative component of the P waves in leads V_{1-2} is broad and deep. The term "P-mitrale" is used to describe left atrial enlargement (hypertrophy) due to mitral stenosis. The diagnostic criteria of left atrial enlargement are summarized elsewhere (*see* Case 33).

A 63-year-old man with COPD was examined at the pulmonary clinic during a periodic checkup.

1. What is the ECG diagnosis?

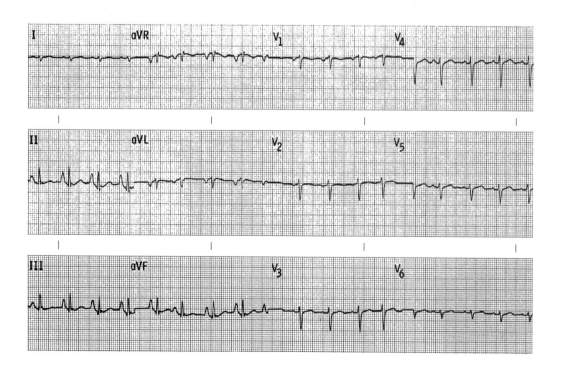

Diagnosis

The underlying cardiac rhythm is sinus tachycardia, with a rate of 105 beats per minute. There are frequent APCs.

The diagnosis of right atrial hypertrophy (enlargement) is made on the basis of tent-shaped and tall P waves in leads II, III, and aVF. The term, "P-pulmonale" is used to describe RAH in patients with COPD. The diagnostic criteria of RAH are summarized as follows:

Diagnostic Criteria of RAH

1. Tent-shaped and tall (3 mm or more) P waves in leads II, III, and aVF.
2. (Less commonly) positive (upright) component of P waves in leads $V_{1,2}$ with amplitude of 2 mm or more.

Another abnormality in this ECG tracing is RVH, which is diagnosed on the basis of right axis deviation with posterior axis deviation of the QRS complexes. The diagnostic criteria of RVH are summarized as follows:

Diagnostic Criteria of RVH

1. Right axis deviation.
2. Tall (or relatively tall) R wave in lead V_1.
3. RR′ pattern in lead V_1.
4. Deep S waves in leads I, aVL, and V_{4-6}.
5. Posterior axis deviation with right axis deviation.
6. Secondary T wave change (strain pattern) in leads V_{1-3} when tall (or relatively tall) R wave or RR′ pattern is present in lead V_1.

By and large, RAH often coexists with RVH in patients with COPD.

A 59-year-old hypertensive male was examined at the cardiac clinic for a periodic medical checkup. The only medication he has been taking was hydrochlorothiazide, 50 mg once daily. He has been relatively asymptomatic except for slight dyspnea on exertion.

1. What is the ECG diagnosis?

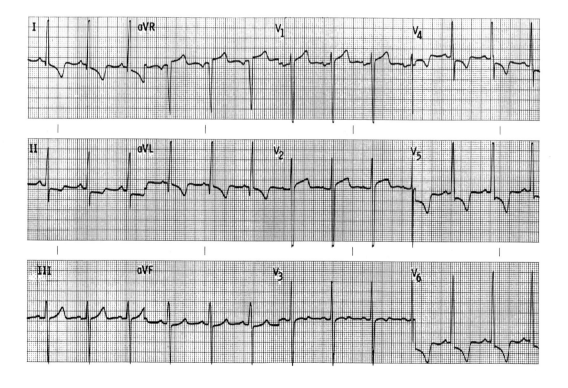

Diagnosis

The cardiac rhythm is sinus, with a rate of 73 beats per minute.

The diagnosis of LVH is established using the conventional diagnostic criteria (see Case 10). Note that the amplitude of the R waves in leads I, aVL, and V_{5-6} is markedly increased, with deep S waves in leads III and V_1. In addition, the secondary T wave change is pronounced in the left precordial leads (so-called left ventricular strain pattern).

Another abnormality in this ECG tracing is left atrial enlargement (see Case 33).

In patients with long-standing hypertension, LVH and LAH often coexist, as seen in this case. Needless to say, the commonest cause of LVH is systemic hypertension.

CASE 47

A 61-year-old woman with a long history of cigarette smoking was seen at the medical clinic for the first time.

    1. What is the ECG diagnosis?

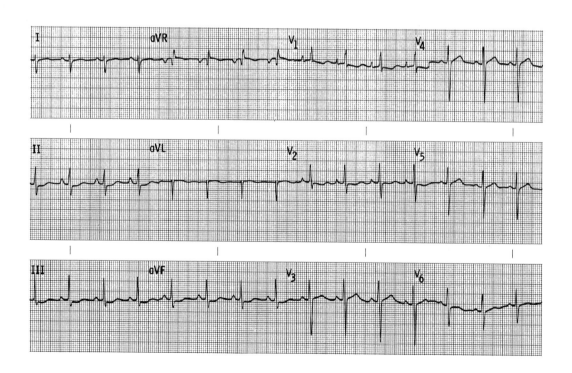

Diagnosis

The cardiac rhythm is sinus, with a rate of 86 beats per minute.

The diagnosis of RVH can be made without much difficulty even by inexperienced readers on the basis of a tall R wave in lead V_1 with right axis deviation of QRS complexes (QRS axis: +120 degrees).

The diagnostic criteria of RVH are summarized elsewhere (*see* Case 45).

In addition, RAH is strongly considered (*see* Case 45).

This woman was found to have advanced COPD, and she was referred to the pulmonary clinic.

CASE 48

This ECG tracing was taken on a 45-year-old man with known RHD. He has been taking digoxin, 0.25 mg daily, for several years.

1. What is the cardiac rhythm diagnosis?
2. What is the ECG diagnosis?

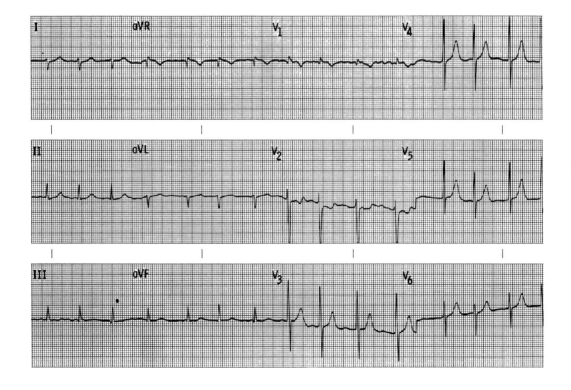

Diagnosis

The cardiac rhythm is AF, with ventricular rate ranging from 78–92 beats per minute.

The diagnosis of RVH is established on the basis of right axis deviation (QRS axis: +110 degrees) with incomplete RBBB pattern (*see* Case 45).

In addition LAH is strongly considered in view of coarse AF (*see* Case 33).

The above-mentioned ECG abnormalities (coarse AF and RVH) are most commonly due to mitral stenosis secondary to RHD.

The patient underwent mitral valve replacement surgery.

CASE 49

A 51-year-old woman was seen at the cardiac clinic for the evaluation of her cardiac status because of various symptoms suggestive of CHF. She was *not* taking any drug.

1. What is the ECG diagnosis?

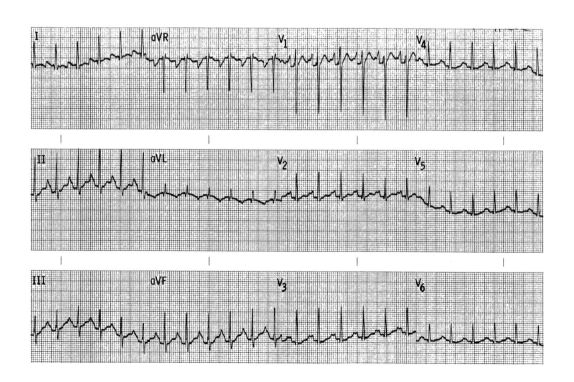

Diagnosis

The cardiac rhythm is sinus tachycardia, with a rate of 135 beats per minute.

It should be noted that the P waves are broad and tall in many limb leads, and the amplitude of both positive as well as negative components of the P wave is increased in lead V_1. Thus the diagnosis of biatrial hypertrophy is strongly considered.

The diagnostic criteria of biatrial hypertrophy are summarized as follows:

Diagnostic Criteria of Biatrial Hypertrophy

1. Wide (3 mm or more) and tall (3 mm or more) P waves in limb leads.

2. Positive (upright) component of P waves in leads $V_{1,2}$, with amplitude of 2 mm or more.

3. Negative (inverted) component of P waves in leads $V_{1,2}$, with depth and width of 1 mm or more.

Cardiomyopathy (idiopathic) was considered to be her underlying cardiac disease.

CASE 50

A 62-year-old hypertensive woman who had suffered a heart attack 2 years previously was examined at the cardiac clinic during a periodic checkup. She has been asymptomatic in recent months.

1. What is the ECG diagnosis?

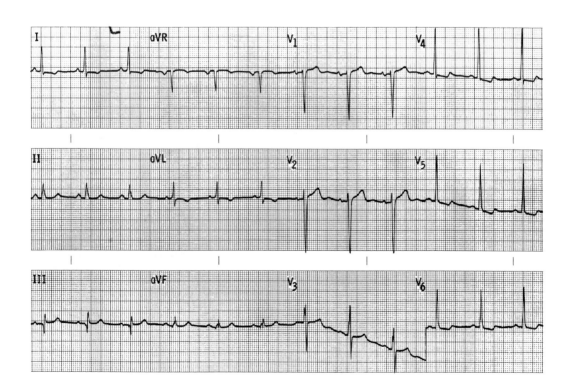

Diagnosis

The cardiac rhythm is sinus, with a rate of 68 beats per minute.

The diagnosis of LVH is established using the conventional criteria (*see* Case 10). In addition, LAH is strongly considered (*see* Case 33).

Another ECG abnormality is old diaphragmatic (inferior) MI (Q waves in leads III and aVF).

Remember that systemic hypertension most commonly produces LVH, and LAH often coexists under this circumstance. Needless to say, hypertension is one of the commonest major risk factors for CAD.

This ECG tracing was obtained from a 43-year-old male with COPD.

1. What is the ECG diagnosis?

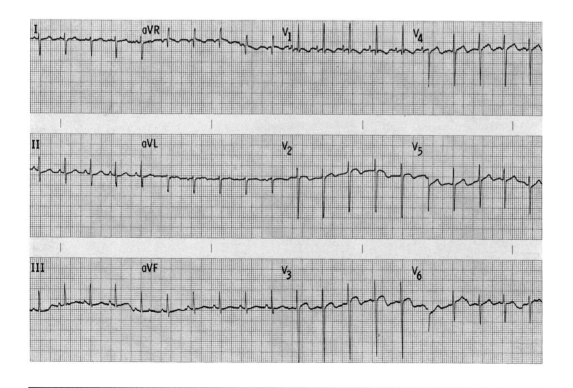

Diagnosis

The cardiac rhythm is sinus tachycardia, with a rate of 118 beats per minute.

The diagnosis of RVH can be established without much difficulty on the basis of right axis deviation of the QRS complexes (axis: +130 degrees) with a tall R wave in lead V_1 (*see* Case 45).

In addition, the P waves are slightly peaked without increased amplitude of the P waves (limb leads and lead V_1). Thus a possibility of RAH is raised (*see* Case 45).

CASE 52

A 70-year-old woman with a long history of hypertension was admitted to the intermediate CCU because of CHF. She has been taking hydrochlorothiazide, 50 mg, only intermittently.

1. What is the cardiac rhythm diagnosis?
2. What is the ECG diagnosis?

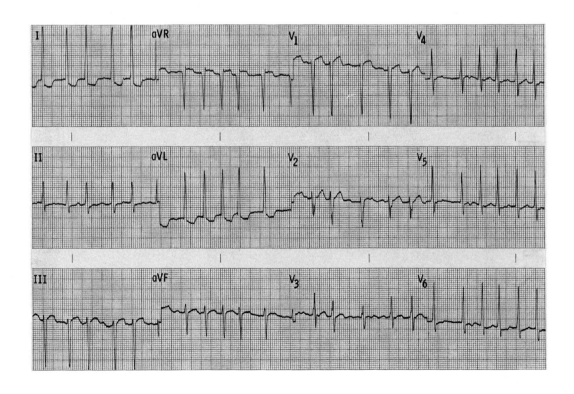

Diagnosis

The cardiac rhythm is AF, with rapid ventricular response (rate: 130–160 beats per minute).

The diagnosis of LVH is established using the conventional criteria (*see* Case 10).

She was rapidly digitalized with continuous diuretic therapy.

By and large, sinus rhythm is unlikely to be restored after digitalization in elderly individuals or in patients with long-standing AF because the majority of these patients have advanced disease in the atria with significant dysfunction in the sinus node (SSS).

This ECG tracing was obtained from a 60-year-old woman with known RHD. She has been taking digoxin, 0.25 mg daily, for several years.

1. What is the cardiac rhythm diagnosis?
2. What is the ECG diagnosis?

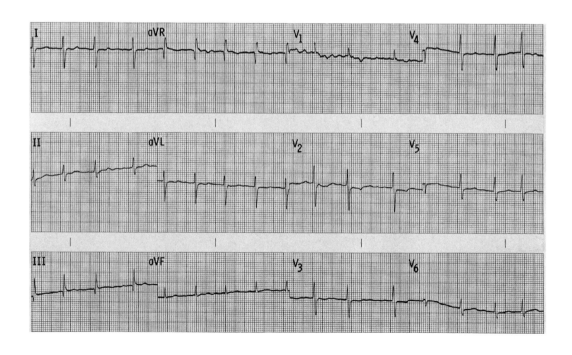

Diagnosis

The cardiac rhythm is AF, with a well-controlled ventricular rate (ranging from 70–95 beats per minute).

The diagnosis of RVH can be established even by inexperienced readers using the conventional criteria (see Case 45), namely, RVH is diagnosed on the basis of a tall R wave in lead V_1 with right axis deviation of the QRS complexes (axis: +125 degrees).

In addition, coarse AF strongly suggests LAH (see Case 33).

The underlying cardiac lesion is almost always mitral stenosis when dealing with any patient showing coarse AF with RVH.

This ECG tracing, which was recorded from a 25-year-old man, was discussed during a weekly ECG conference because the ECG finding was considered to be very unusual for the patient's age. He never had a complete medical evaluation previously.

1. What is the ECG diagnosis?
2. What is most likely the underlying heart disease?

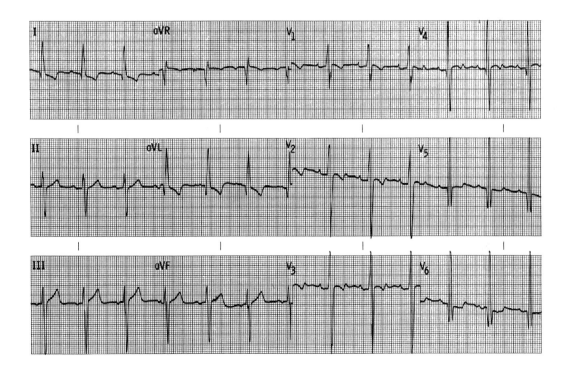

Diagnosis

The cardiac rhythm is sinus, with a rate of 70 beats per minute.

The first ECG abnormality in this tracing is left anterior hemiblock (the QRS axis: −50 degrees). The diagnostic criteria of left anterior hemiblock are summarized elsewhere (*see* Case 27).

The next ECG abnormality is LVH (*see* Case 10). In addition, LAH is diagnosed (*see* Case 33).

The most interesting ECG findings in this tracing include a tall R wave in lead V_1 and deep Q waves in leads V_{5-6}. This ECG abnormality is considered to be due to ventricular septal hypertrophy.

This young man was found to have IHSS. Posterolateral MI is superficially simulated.

This ECG tracing was obtained from a 62-year-old woman with mild CHF secondary to systemic hypertension. Her medications included digoxin, 0.25 mg, and hydrochlorothiazide, 50 mg, once daily, with one more cardiac drug.

1. What is the cardiac rhythm diagnosis?
2. What is the ECG diagnosis?
3. What cardiac drug is responsible for the production of the somewhat unusual feature of her arrhythmia?

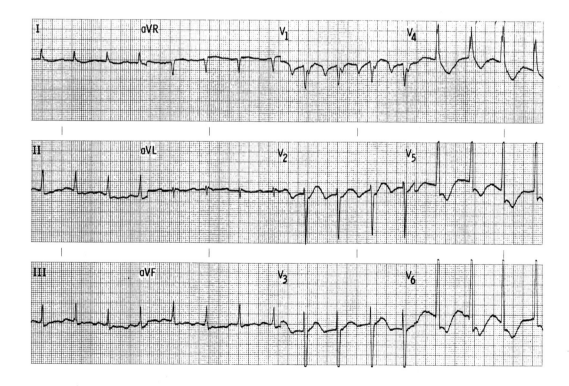

Diagnosis

The cardiac rhythm is atrial flutter (atrial rate: 180 beats per minute), with 2 : 1 A-V response (ventricular rate: 90 beats per minute). Unusually slow atrial flutter is most commonly due to quinidine, and is less commonly due to other quinidine-like drugs such as procainamide. Remember that the usual atrial rates range from 250–350 beats per minute in a pure form of atrial flutter (see Case 20).

The diagnosis of LVH is made using conventional criteria (see Case 10). The QRS duration is diffusely increased as a result of nonspecific (diffuse) intraventricular block. Nonspecific intraventricular block is commonly produced when there is severe LVH, as seen in this case.

Obviously quinidine was responsible for producing an unusually slow atrial flutter cycle in this patient. The flutter waves are best seen in leads V_{1-2}.

A 40-year-old woman with known sarcoidosis was seen at the pulmonary clinic during a periodic medical checkup.

   1. What is the ECG diagnosis?

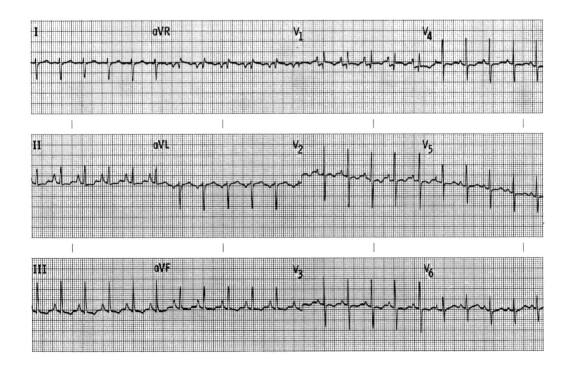

Diagnosis

The cardiac rhythm is sinus tachycardia, with a rate of 128 beats per minute.

The diagnosis of RVH can be made without much difficulty on the basis of a tall R wave in lead V_1, with right axis deviation of QRS complexes (QRS axis: +120 degrees). The diagnostic criteria of RVH are summarized elsewhere (see Case 45).

In addition, tall and peaking P waves in leads II, III, aVF, and V_1 are indicative of RAH (P-pulmonale, see Case 45).

It is not uncommon to observe a small Q wave in lead V_1 (sometimes in leads V_{1-3}) in severe RVH.

CASE 57

The ECG tracing was obtained from a 51-year-old woman with known CAD associated with COPD.

   1. What is the ECG diagnosis?

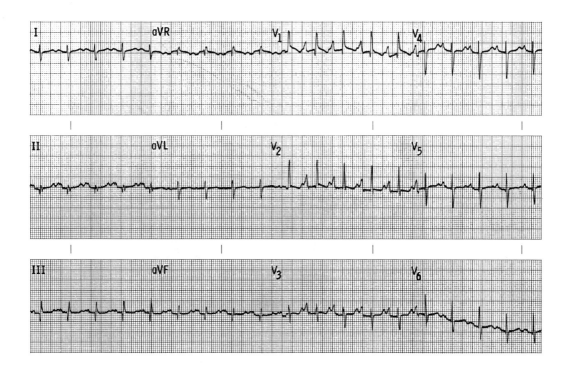

Diagnosis

The cardiac rhythm is sinus tachycardia, with a rate of 110 beats per minute, and first degree A-V block.

The diagnosis of RVH is established on the basis of tall R waves in leads V_{1-2}, with right axis deviation of the QRS complexes (QRS axis: +125 degrees).

Another ECG abnormality is biatrial hypertrophy (see Case 49). Note that the P waves are broad and notched in many limb leads, and the P waves are tall in leads V_{1-3}.

In addition, old diaphragmatic (inferior) MI can be diagnosed without any difficulty on the basis of Q waves in leads II, III, and aVF.

Digitalis intoxication was suspected in a 51-year-old woman with long-standing CHF. She has been taking digoxin, 0.25 mg, and hydrochlorothiazide, 50 mg, once daily.

1. What is the cardiac rhythm diagnosis?
2. What is the ECG diagnosis?

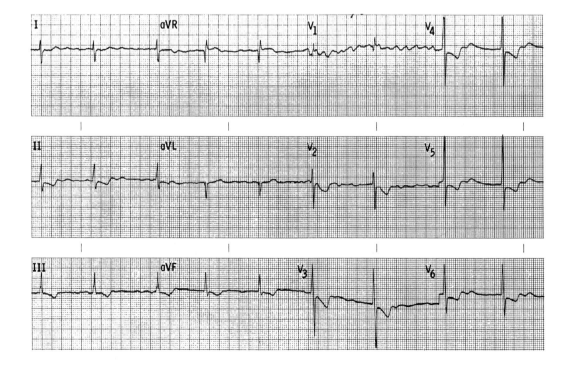

Diagnosis

The underlying cardiac rhythm is AF. The ventricular rate is very slow (45 beats per minute) as a result of advanced A-V block. In addition, some RR intervals are constant (regular) because of intermittent A-V JEB.

The diagnosis of biventricular hypertrophy can be entertained on the basis of right axis deviation of the QRS complexes (QRS axis: +125 degrees), incomplete RBBB pattern (or relatively tall R wave) in lead V_1, and increased amplitude of R waves in leads V_{5-6}. The diagnostic criteria of biventricular hypertrophy are summarized below:

Diagnostic Criteria of Biventricular Hypertrophy

1. LVH pattern in the precordial leads and right axis deviation.
2. Tall (or relatively tall) R waves in all precordial leads.
3. Katz-Wachtel phenomenon.
4. P-pulmonale or P-congenitale in limb leads and LVH pattern in the precordial leads.

Another ECG abnormality is prominent U waves (best shown in leads V_{4-6}), indicative of hypokalemia.

The patient's cardiac arrhythmia is considered to be due to DI. Hypokalemia often predisposes to DI.

A 23-year-old man with known congenital heart disease was referred to a cardiac surgeon for repair of his cardiac lesion.

1. What is the ECG diagnosis?
2. What is most likely the underlying cardiac lesion?

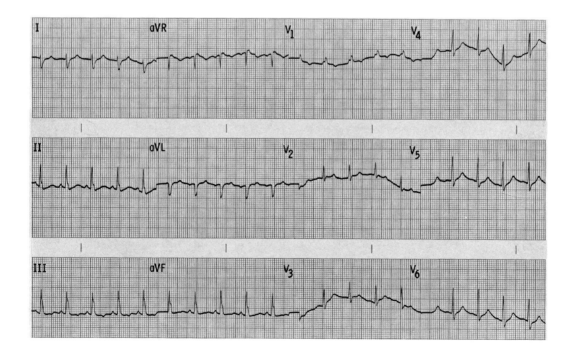

Diagnosis

The cardiac rhythm is sinus tachycardia, with a rate of 114 beats per minute.

The diagnosis of incomplete RBBB can be entertained using conventional diagnostic criteria (*see* Case 34).

RVH is strongly considered because of coexisting right axis deviation of the QRS complexes (QRS axis: +105 degrees).

It has been shown that ASD is most commonly associated with RBBB (often incomplete RBBB) among all congenital cardiac anomalies combined. In ostium secundum type of ASD, the QRS axis may be normal, or it may show right axis deviation, as seen in this case. On the other hand, ostium primum defect almost always produces left anterior hemiblock in the presence of RBBB.

It can be said that the diagnosis of ASD is extremely unlikely when ECG demonstrates no evidence of RBBB (complete or incomplete).

This ECG tracing was obtained from a 60-year-old woman with RHD.

    She has been taking digoxin, 0.25 mg daily, for several years.

1. What is the cardiac rhythm diagnosis?
2. What is the ECG diagnosis?

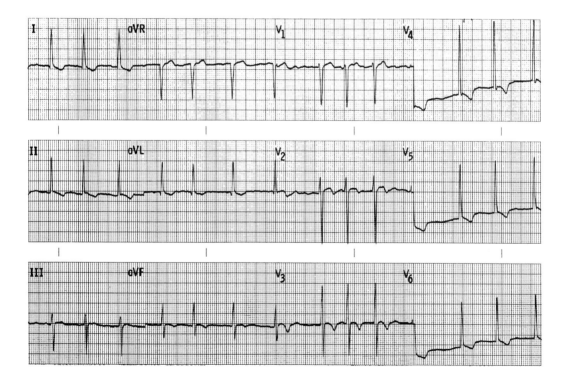

Diagnosis

The cardiac rhythm is AF, with ideal ventricular rate (70–80 beats per minute).

The diagnosis of LVH is established on the basis of tall R waves in leads I, aVL, and V_{5-6} and deep S waves in leads III and V_1 associated with secondary T wave change in the left precordial leads. The di- agnostic criteria of LVH are found elsewhere (see Case 10).

This patient was found to have aortic stenosis. It has been shown that severe aortic stenosis is often associated with inverted T waves involving practically all precordial leads.

CASE 61

A 76-year-old man with known COPD was seen at the pulmonary clinic during a periodic medical checkup. A cardiologist was consulted in the evaluation of his arrhythmia.

1. What is the cardiac rhythm diagnosis?
2. What is the ECG diagnosis?

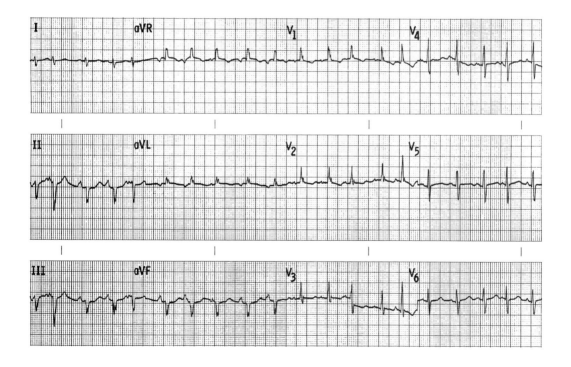

Diagnosis

The underlying cardiac rhythm is sinus tachycardia (rate: 103 beats per minute), but there are frequent APCs with atrial group beats. Some APCs show aberrant ventricular conduction.

The diagnosis of RVH can be made on the basis of incomplete RBBB pattern in lead V_1, with right axis deviation of the QRS complexes (*see* Case 45).

In addition, tall and peaked P waves in leads II, III, and aVF are diagnostic of RAH (P-pulmonale).

Another ECG abnormality in this tracing is marked superior axis deviation of the QRS complex, indicative of left anterior hemiblock (*see* Case 27). The QRS axis in this ECG tracing is calculated to be −90 degrees, namely, this markedly superior and vertical QRS axis shift is due to two independent factors, including left anterior hemiblock and RVH.

CASE 62

A 46-year-old man was evaluated at the cardiac clinic because of heart murmurs. He gave a history of rheumatic fever in the past but has been relatively healthy otherwise.

1. What is the cardiac rhythm diagnosis?
2. What is the ECG diagnosis?

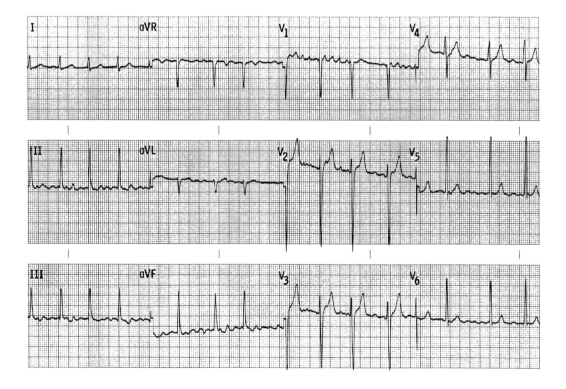

Diagnosis

The cardiac rhythm is atrial flutter-fibrillation (a mixed form of AF and flutter) or coarse AF.

LAH is strongly considered when dealing with coarse AF.

Amplitude of the R waves in leads V_{5-6} is markedly increased, with a deep S wave in lead V_1. This ECG finding meets the criteria of LVH (see Case 10) except that the secondary T wave change (so-called "strain pattern") is not present. Thus the diagnosis of diastolic overloading LVH is made.

This patient was found to have aortic insufficiency, mitral insufficiency, and mitral stenosis as manifestations of RHD.

CASE 63

This ECG tracing was obtained from a 64-year-old woman with known RHD. She has been taking digoxin, 0.25 mg, daily.

1. What is the cardiac rhythm diagnosis?
2. What is the ECG diagnosis?

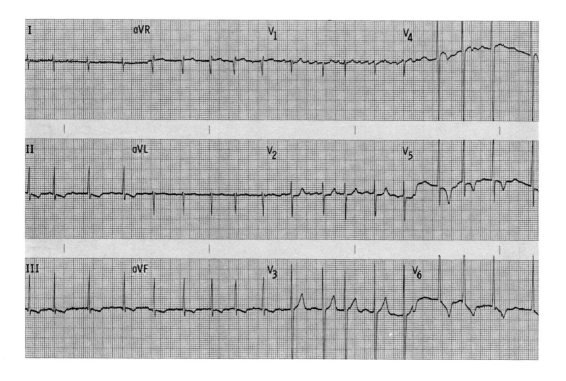

Diagnosis

The cardiac rhythm is atrial flutter-fibrillation, with a relatively well-controlled ventricular rate (85–100 beats per minute).

The diagnosis of biventricular hypertrophy can be entertained on the basis of right axis deviation of the QRS complexes (QRS axis: +105 degrees) in the presence of LVH in the precordial leads. The diagnostic criteria of biventricular hypertrophy are summarized in Case 58.

This patient was found to have aortic stenosis and mitral stenosis as manifestations of RHD. Atrial flutter-fibrillation or coarse AF suggests LAH (*see* Case 33).

CHAPTER THREE

HEMIBLOCKS, BUNDLE BRANCH BLOCK, BIFASCICULAR BLOCK, AND TRIFASCICULAR BLOCK

CASE 64

A 69-year-old woman was admitted to the CCU via the ER because of severe chest pain of a few hours duration. She had not been taking any drug before this admission and had been relatively healthy, otherwise.

1. What is the ECG diagnosis?
2. Is an artificial cardiac pacemaker indicated?

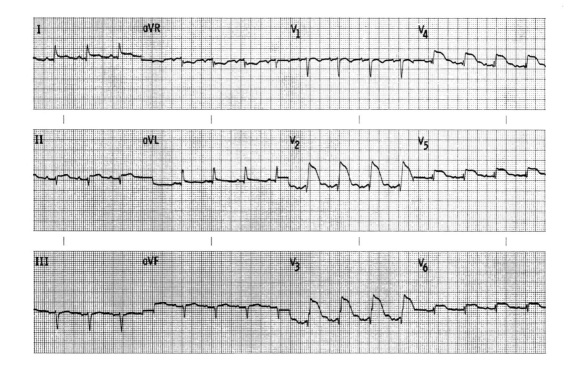

Diagnosis

The rhythm is sinus, with a rate of 95 beats per minute.

Acute extensive anterior MI is diagnosed on the basis of Q waves and/or marked reduction of the R wave amplitude in the entire precordial leads associated with marked ST segment elevation. A similar ECG finding is observed in leads I and aVL, indicating high lateral wall involvement of the left ventricle.

Another ECG abnormality is left anterior hemiblock (*see* Case 27).

The prophylactic artificial pacing is *not* indicated for left anterior hemiblock even if it is due to acute anterior MI.

CASE 65

This is a routine ECG tracing obtained from a 61-year-old apparently healthy man.

    1. What is the ECG diagnosis?

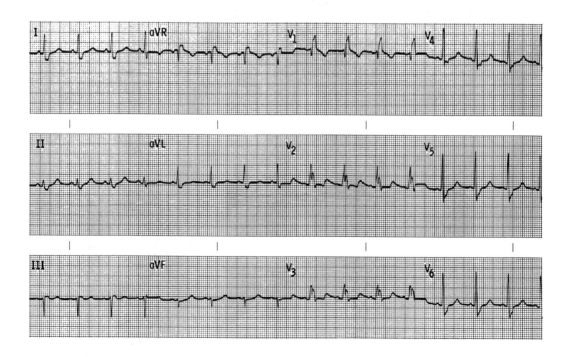

Diagnosis

The cardiac rhythm is sinus, with a rate of 88 beats per minute.

The diagnosis of RBBB can be made even by inexperienced readers using the conventional diagnostic criteria (*see* Case 34). Note RR' pattern (M-shaped) of the QRS complexes in leads V_{1-3}, with deep and slurred S waves in leads I, aVL, and V_{4-6} as a result of delayed right ven-tricular activation. In addition the secondary T wave change is observed in leads V_{1-3} as a manifestation of RBBB.

It has been shown that RBBB may be found in healthy people, and the presence of RBBB is *not* indicative of any organic heart disease. On the other hand, many cardiac patients may show RBBB.

CASE 66

This ECG tracing was taken on a 58-year-old hypertensive man.

1. What is the ECG diagnosis?

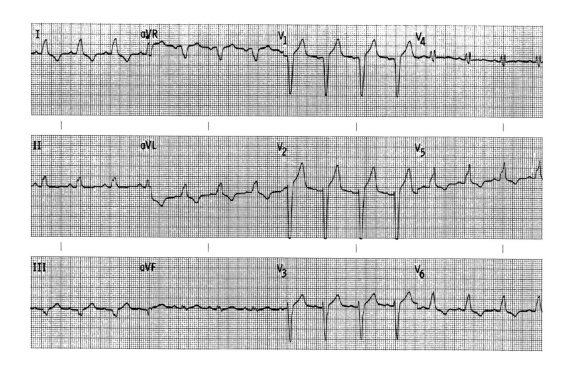

Diagnosis

The cardiac rhythm is sinus, with a rate of 87 beats per minute.

The diagnosis of LBBB can be established without any difficulty using the conventional diagnostic criteria (*see* Case 33). Note that the left precordial leads reveal broad R waves or M-shaped pattern of the QRS complexes associated with secondary T wave change. The most important sign of LBBB is the absence of small Q waves (septal Q waves) in the left precordial leads because of reversed initial activation of the ventricular septum.

Clinically LBBB is most commonly encountered in patients with systemic hypertension. The next commonest cause of LBBB is probably aortic stenosis. Less commonly LBBB may be observed in patients with CAD and cardiomyopathies. By and large LBBB is very unusual in healthy individuals.

This ECG tracing was obtained from a 50-year-old woman with multiple risk factors (eg, obesity, hypertension, diabetes mellitus, cigarette smoking, and family history of CAD) for CAD. She was admitted to the CCU because of a heart attack. Soon after this ECG tracing was recorded, she developed BFB consisting of RBBB and left anterior hemiblock. Later the cardiac rhythm changed to 2 : 1 A-V block in the presence of BFB.

1. What is the ECG diagnosis?
2. Is permanent artificial pacing indicated?

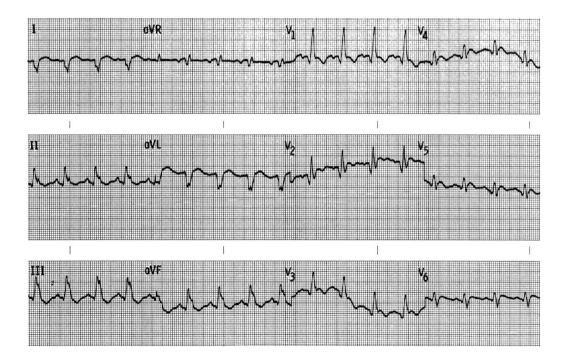

Diagnosis

The cardiac rhythm is sinus, with a rate of 100 beats per minute.

There are many different ECG abnormalities. The first ECG abnormality is recent extensive anterior MI (abnormal Q waves in all precordial leads associated with ST segment elevation). The second abnormality is old diaphragmatic (inferior) MI, manifested by Q waves in leads II, III, and aVF. The third ECG abnormality is BFB, which consists of RBBB and left posterior hemiblock (QRS axis: +120 degrees).

As indicated earlier, this patient developed RBBB with left anterior hemiblock and intermittent 2 : 1 A-V block. When these ECG abnormalities are interpreted together, this patient definitely shows evidence of advanced BBBB. Thus a permanent artificial pacemaker is indicated. The diagnostic criteria of BBBB are summarized in Case 7.

CASE 68

This ECG tracing was obtained from a 59-year-old man with known CAD.

1. What is the ECG diagnosis?

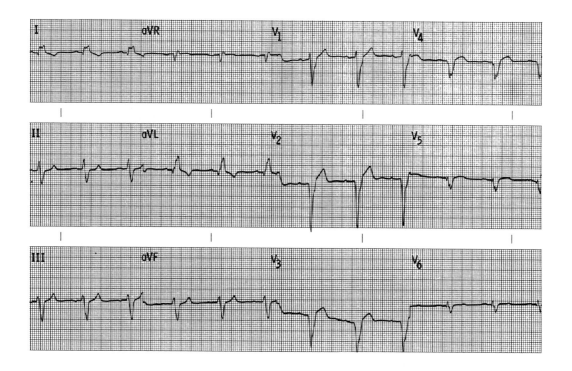

Diagnosis

The cardiac rhythm is sinus, with a rate of 68 beats per minute.

Extensive anterior MI (except septum) is diagnosed on the basis of QS waves or Q waves in leads V_{2-6}.

Another ECG abnormality is left anterior hemiblock, manifested by marked left axis deviation of the QRS complexes (QRS axis: -55 degrees). In addition, the QRS complexes are very broad, indicative of nonspecific (diffuse) intraventricular block.

LBBB is superficially simulated (*see* Case 33).

A 47-year-old man with a long history of cigarette smoking was admitted to CCU via the ER because a heart attack was suspected.

1. What is the ECG diagnosis?
2. Is the prophylactic artificial pacing indicated?

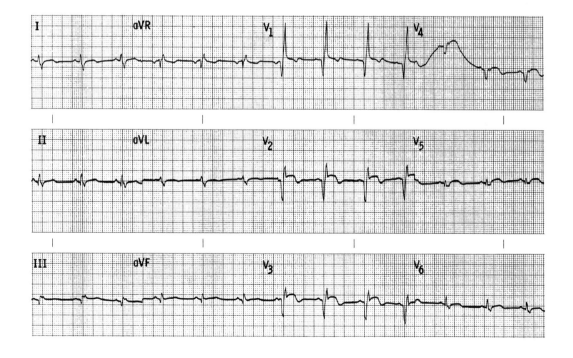

Diagnosis

The cardiac rhythm is sinus, with a rate of 74 beats per minute.

The diagnosis of acute extensive anterior MI can be established on the basis of Q waves in the entire precordial leads, with ST segment elevation and T wave inversion.

Another ECG abnormality is old diaphragmatic (inferior) MI (Q waves in leads II, III, and aVF).

In addition, the diagnosis of RBBB can be established using the conventional criteria (see Case 34). The typical RBBB pattern is altered in this tracing simply because of the coexisting anterior MI.

The prophylactic artificial pacing is generally *not* indicated for RBBB even if acute anterior MI is a direct cause of RBBB.

This ECG tracing was taken on a 55-year-old man who was admitted to the CCU.

1. What is the ECG diagnosis?
2. Is the prophylactic artificial pacing indicated?

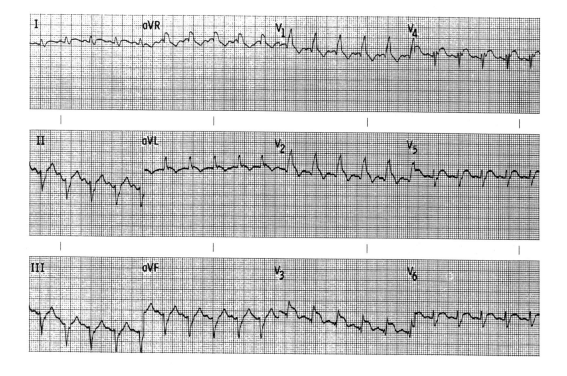

Diagnosis

The cardiac rhythm is sinus tachycardia, with a rate of 128 beats per minute. There is an APC (the tenth beat).

Acute anteroseptal MI is diagnosed on the basis of pathologic Q waves in leads V_{1-3} associated with marked ST segment elevation and T wave inversion.

Another ECG abnormality is BFB, which consists of RBBB and left anterior hemiblock (the QRS axis: −85 degrees).

The prophylactic artificial pacing is highly recommended for BFB of acute onset as a result of acute anteroseptal MI.

This is a routine ECG tracing obtained from
an 86-year-old woman.

    1. What is the ECG diagnosis?

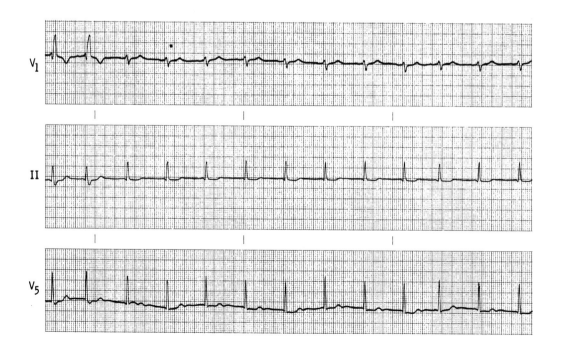

Diagnosis

The cardiac rhythm is slight sinus arrhythmia, with a rate of 78 beats per minute.

There are two bizarre beats (first two beats), which represent an intermittent RBBB. RBBB occurs when the heart rate is slightly faster. Thus RBBB in this tracing is "rate dependent." Intermittent RBBB has no clinical significance, but the finding superficially resembles VPCs. The diagnostic criteria of RBBB are found in Case 34.

Intermittent RBBB becomes eventually fixed RBBB later.

Posterior MI is a remote possibility in view of a relatively tall R wave in lead V_1 with upright T wave.

This ECG tracing, which belongs to a 71-year-old man, was discussed during a weekly advanced ECG conference because of somewhat unusual features of the trac-ing. He had suffered from a heart attack 2 months previously.

1. What is the ECG diagnosis?

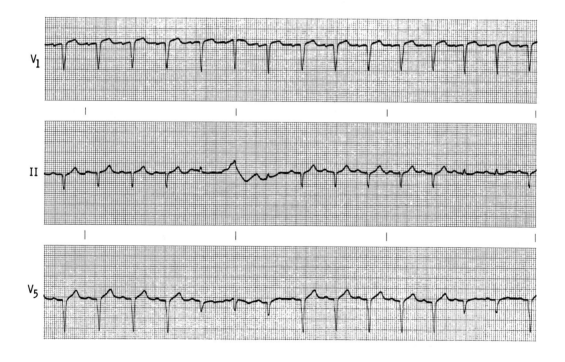

Diagnosis

The cardiac rhythm is sinus, with a rate of 92 beats per minute.

There are two kinds of the QRS complexes. Note that there is an artifact in the midportion of the tracing (lead II). He had suffered from extensive anterior MI (QS waves in the entire precordial leads), and there is a possibility of old diaphragmatic MI (only leads V_1, II, and V_5 are shown here).

Some experienced readers may be able to diagnose intermittent left anterior hemiblock, which causes two kinds of QRS complexes. Deep S waves in leads II and V_5 are due to intermittent left anterior hemiblock. Intermittent left anterior hemiblock in this tracing is *not* related to the heart rate change. Therefore this finding represents "rate independent" left anterior hemiblock.

Clinically, intermittent left anterior hemiblock is insignificant, but this ECG finding superficially simulates intermittent slow VT (idioventricular tachycardia, accelerated idioventricular rhythm, or nonparoxysmal VT).

This ECG tracing was taken on a 79-year-old man during his annual medical check-up. He was asymptomatic.

1. What is the ECG diagnosis?
2. Is an artificial pacemaker indicated?

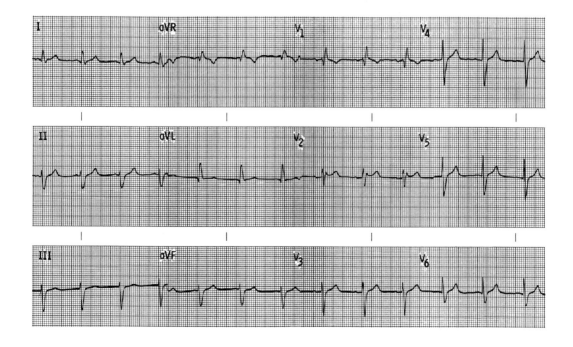

Diagnosis

The cardiac rhythm is sinus, with a rate of 72 beats per minute.

The diagnosis of BFB consisting of RBBB and left anterior hemiblock can be readily made using the conventional criteria (*see* Case 7). Remember that a combination of RBBB and left anterior hemiblock is the commonest form of BBBB.

Artificial pacing is *not* indicated for asymptomatic and chronic BFB.

CASE 74

This ECG tracing was obtained from a 54-year-old woman with no evidence of apparent heart disease.

1. What is the ECG diagnosis?

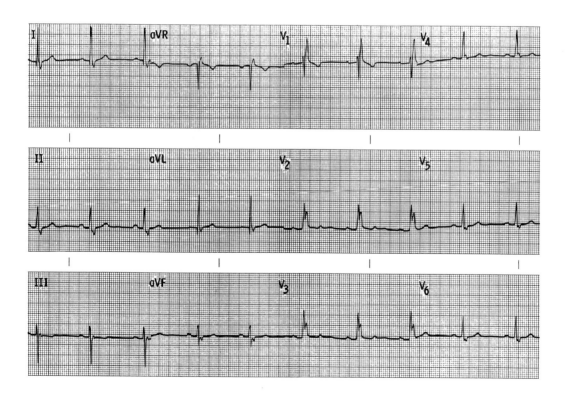

Diagnosis

The cardiac rhythm is mild sinus bradycardia, with a rate of 57 beats per minute.

The diagnosis of RBBB can be made without any difficulty even by inexperienced readers using the conventional diagnostic criteria (*see* Case 34). As discussed earlier, RBBB is occasionally found in apparently healthy individuals.

A possibility of LVH is raised on the basis of increased amplitude of the R waves in leads I and aVL, with deep S wave in lead III.

CASE 75

This ECG tracing, which was obtained from an 81-year-old woman, was discussed during a weekly ECG conference in the evaluation of various QRS complexes.

1. What is the ECG diagnosis?

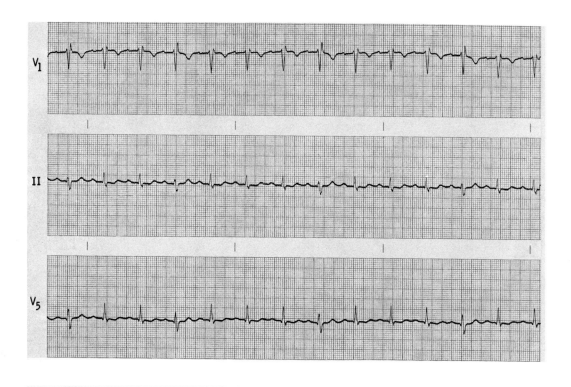

Diagnosis

The cardiac rhythm is sinus, with a rate of 83 beats per minute, and there is first degree A-V block (the PR interval: 0.22 second).

It is interesting to note that the configuration of the QRS complexes varies although every beat reveals RBBB pattern. Thus this ECG tracing demonstrates RBBB of a varying degree, meaning that the degree of RBBB varies from beat to beat.

In addition, left anterior hemiblock occurs intermittently.

When the above-mentioned ECG findings are interpreted together, intermittent BFB can be diagnosed.

A possibility of anterolateral MI is raised because of Q wave in lead V_5.

CASE 76

This ECG tracing was obtained from an 82-year-old man with chronic CHF. He has been taking digoxin, 0.25 mg daily, for several years. He denied any history of fainting or near syncope.

1. What is the cardiac rhythm diagnosis?
2. What is the ECG diagnosis?
3. Is an artificial pacemaker indicated?

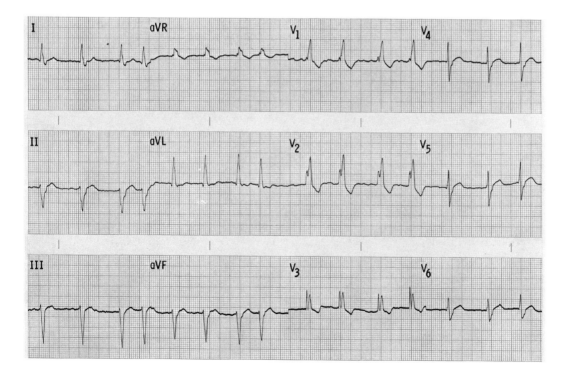

Diagnosis

The cardiac rhythm is AF, with ventricular rates ranging from 78–100 beats per minute. Some RR intervals are regular because of intermittent nonparoxysmal A-V JT (eg, the first three beats).

The diagnosis of BFB consisting of RBBB and left anterior hemiblock (the QRS axis: −75 degrees) can be established using the conventional diagnostic criteria (*see* Case 7).

Artificial pacing is *not* indicated for chronic BFB as long as there is no evidence of a more advanced form of BBBB (eg, intermittent Mobitz type II A-V block or intermittent VER).

This is a routine ECG tracing obtained from a 77-year-old woman with no apparent cardiac disease.

    1. What is the ECG diagnosis?

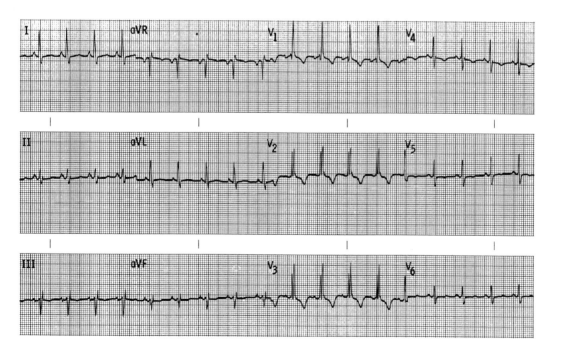

Diagnosis

The cardiac rhythm is sinus tachycardia, with a rate of 104 beats per minute.

The diagnosis of incomplete RBBB can be made by using the conventional diagnostic criteria (*see* Case 34). Note RR′ (M-shaped QRS complex) in leads V_{1-3}, with slurred S waves in leads I and V_{4-6}. The secondary T wave change is shown in leads V_{1-3}. The QRS duration of 0.10 second.

Incomplete RBBB is insignificant clinically.

CASE 78

This ECG tracing, which belongs to an 81-year-old woman, was discussed during a weekly student ECG conference.

1. What is the ECG diagnosis?

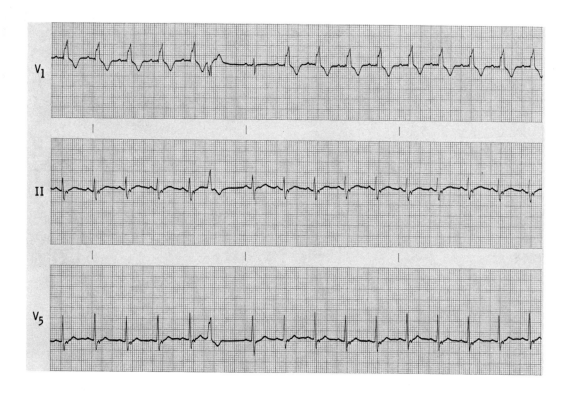

Diagnosis

The cardiac rhythm is sinus, with a rate of 100 beats per minute.

There are three kinds of QRS complexes. The first bizarre beat (the sixth beat) represents a VPC. A normal (narrow) QRS complex immediately following a VPC is normally a conducted sinus beat (the seventh beat). The remaining QRS complexes demonstrate RBBB.

When the above ECG findings are interpreted together, this patient shows intermittent RBBB, which is rate dependent. Specifically, she has "tachycardia-dependent" RBBB. In other words, her right bundle branch system is able to function normally when the heart rate is slower than 70 beats per minute.

Intermittent RBBB is insignificant clinically, but some inexperienced readers may find some difficulty in interpreting this finding correctly.

CASE 79

This ECG tracing was taken on an 80-year-old woman.

1. What is the cardiac rhythm diagnosis?
2. What is the ECG diagnosis?

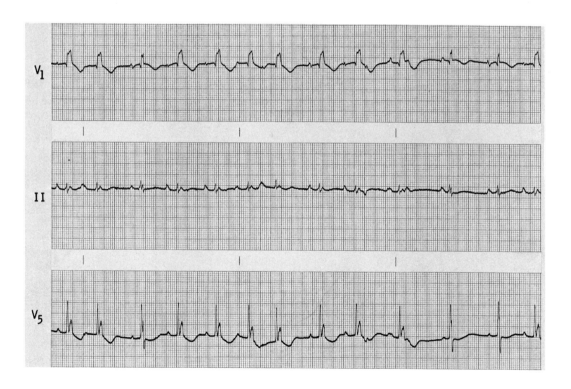

Diagnosis

The underlying cardiac rhythm is sinus, but there are frequent APCs with group beats.

There are two kinds of QRS complexes because complete and incomplete RBBB occur intermittently. Her intermittent complete and incomplete RBBB is *not* exactly rate dependent, although incomplete RBBB is generally observed during slower heart rate.

CASE 80

This is a routine ECG tracing obtained from a healthy 30-year-old woman.

1. What is the ECG diagnosis?

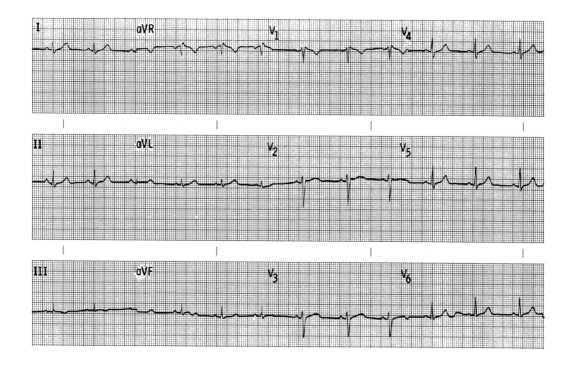

Diagnosis

The cardiac rhythm is sinus arrhythmia, with rates ranging from 70–78 beats per minute.

The diagnosis of incomplete RBBB can be made by most readers using conventional criteria (*see* Case 34). This minimum degree of incomplete RBBB is considered to be a normal variant.

These two ECG tracings (**A** and **B**) were obtained from a 76-year-old man on two different occasions (two days apart).

1. What is the cardiac rhythm diagnosis?

2. What is the ECG diagnosis?
3. What is the proper therapeutic approach?

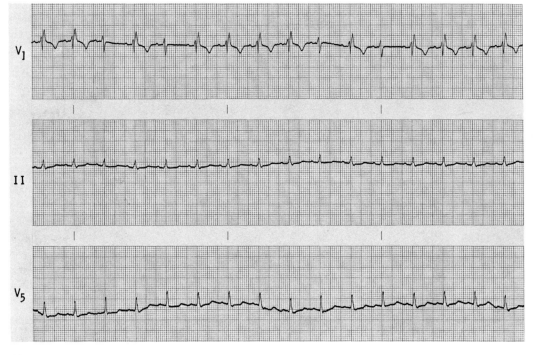

A

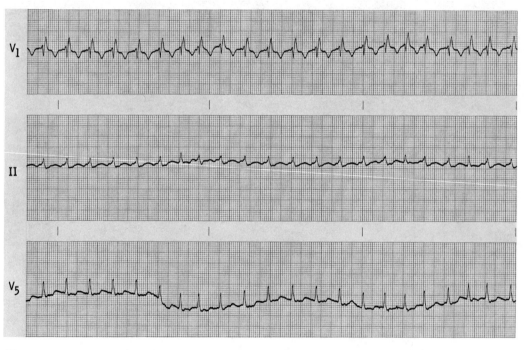

B

Diagnosis

Tracing A:

The cardiac rhythm is sinus, with a rate of 100 beats per minute. There are two kinds of QRS complexes because of intermittent RBBB. Frequent VPCs or even short runs of VT are superficially simulated.

Tracing B:

Two days later the cardiac rhythm had changed to atrial flutter-fibrillation, with rapid ventricular response (ventricular rate: 130–155 beats per minute). In this tracing RBBB persists throughout.

The drug of choice for AF or atrial flutter-fibrillation with rapid ventricular response is rapid digitalization.

CHAPTER FOUR

ATRIOVENTRICULAR BLOCK

This ECG tracing, which belongs to an 82-year-old man, was presented to the professor teaching rounds because of its educational value for medical students and house officers. Digitalis toxicity was suspected.

1. What is the cardiac rhythm diagnosis?

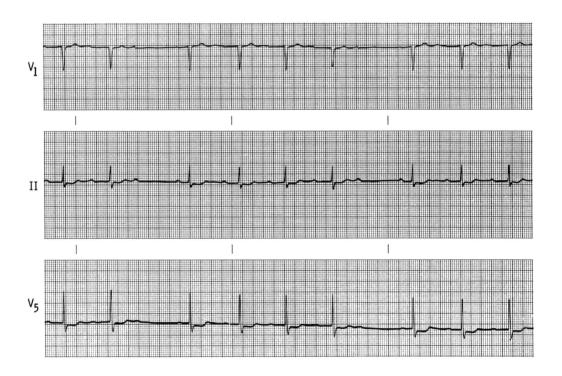

V_1

II

V_5

Diagnosis

The cardiac rhythm is sinus (atrial rate: 70 beats per minute), with 5 : 4 Wenckebach A-V block (ventricular rate: 56 beats per minute).

The characteristic features of Wenckebach A-V block include progressive lengthening of PR intervals, with progressive shortening of the RR intervals until a blocked P wave occurs. The progressive shortening of the RR intervals is observed during Wenckebach A-V block because the degree of increment in the PR interval prolongation becomes progressively less until a blocked P wave occurs.

The A-V conduction ratio is expressed in Wenckebach A-V block with the numbers of the P waves versus the numbers of the QRS complexes. For instance, 5 : 4 Wenckebach A-V block is diagnosed, as seen in this tracing when four of five P waves are conducted to the ventricles, meaning five P waves versus four QRS complexes.

By and large, Wenckebach A-V block is most commonly due to two cardiac disorders, including digitalis toxicity and acute diaphragmatic MI (*see* Cases 83, 87, 88, 90, and 98).

Wenckebach A-V block (Mobitz type I A-V block) nearly always represents A-V nodal block (block within the A-V junction). On the other hand, Mobitz type II A-V block represents infranodal block (block distal to A-V junction, *see* Case 91). In general, Wenckebach A-V block is a transient phenomenon, whereas Mobitz type II A-V block is irreversible.

CASE 83

A 46-year-old man was admitted to the CCU because of recent heart attack. The ECG tracings taken on other occasions are shown elsewhere.

1. What is the cardiac rhythm diagnosis?

2. What is the ECG diagnosis?
3. What is the proper therapeutic approach to his cardiac arrhythmia?

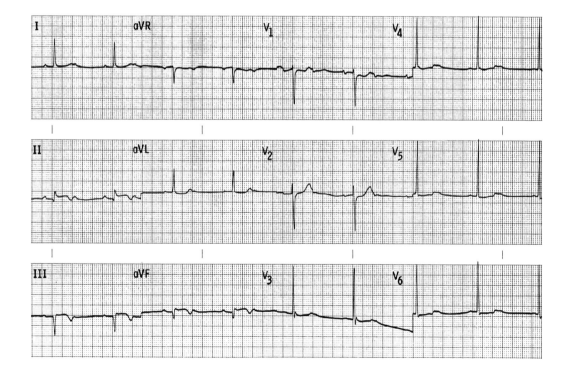

Diagnosis

The cardiac rhythm is sinus (atrial rate: 100 beats per minute), with 2 : 1 A-V block (ventricular rate: 50 beats per minute). When dealing with 2 : 1 A-V block with normal QRS complexes, especially in patients with acute diaphragmatic MI, the block is a variant of Wenckebach A-V block (see Cases 87 and 98).

The diagnosis of acute diaphragmatic MI can be established without any difficulty on the basis of pathologic Q waves in leads II, III, and aVF, associated with ST segment elevation and T wave inversion. In addition, this ECG tracing reveals LVH (see Case 10).

As indicated earlier (see Case 82), Wenckebach A-V block (including 2 : 1 A-V block) in acute diaphragmatic MI is almost always a transient phenomenon and is self-limited. Thus no active treatment is necessary for this patient's arrhythmia as long as the arrhythmia produces no significant symptom or hemodynamic abnormality.

This ECG tracing, obtained from a 73-year-old man, was discussed during a weekly ECG conference. He denied any episode of syncope and near syncope.

1. What is the cardiac rhythm diagnosis?
2. What is the proper therapeutic approach?

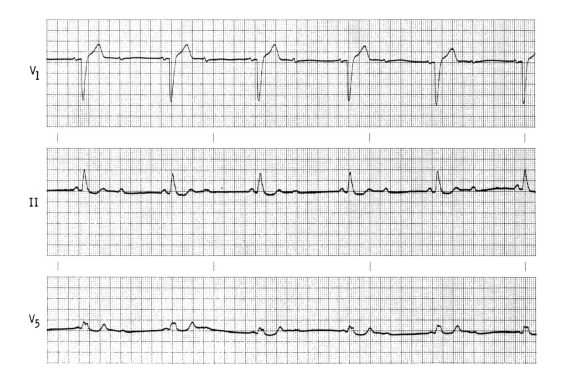

Diagnosis

The cardiac rhythm is sinus (atrial rate: 70 beats per minute), with 2 : 1 A-V block (ventricular rate: 35 beats per minute). Although the type of A-V block *cannot* be determined with certainty when 2 : 1 A-V block persists, the A-V block is almost always a variant of Mobitz type II A-V block when the conducted beats show RBBB, LBBB, hemiblock, or BFB, as shown in this tracing. Thus A-V block under this circumstance represents infranodal block, which is usually irreversible.

Permanent artificial cardiac pacing should be strongly considered in patients with Mobitz type II A-V block, even if the patient is asymptomatic.

Obviously all conducted sinus beats exhibit LBBB.

CASE 85

Cardiac consultation was requested in the evaluation of the cardiac arrhythmia in a 22-year-old woman with no demonstrable heart disease. She denied any cardiac symptom and was *not* taking any drug.

1. What is the cardiac rhythm diagnosis?
2. What is the proper way to handle this arrhythmia?

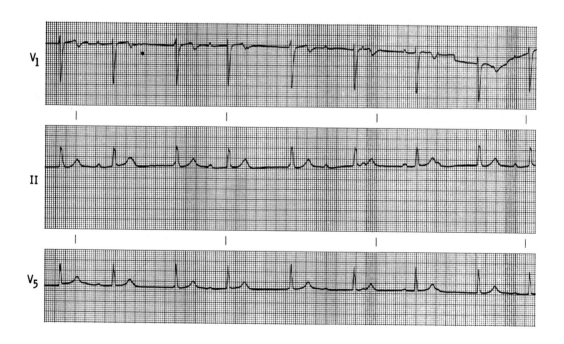

Diagnosis

Inexperienced readers may erroneously diagnose the cardiac rhythm simply as sinus arrhythmia or wandering atrial pacemaker. However, on close observation it becomes obvious that the atrial and ventricular activities are independent in most areas, namely, the RR intervals are regular and slow (rate: 48 beats per minute) in most areas, and intermittently the RR interval is short. The short RR interval occurs intermittently because the sinus impulses are conducted to the ventricles intermittently (the second, fourth, seventh, and ninth beats). The remaining QRS complexes represent A-V JEB.

When the above-mentioned ECG findings are interpreted together, this tracing demonstrates sinus rhythm (atrial rate: 82 beats per minute) with advanced A-V block (the A-V conduction ratio consisting of 3 : 1 and 5 : 1) and intermittent A-V JEBs producing incomplete A-V dissociation. The block in this case is most likely A-V nodal block because all QRS complexes are normal.

Since the patient is entirely asymptomatic, no urgent treatment is necessary. However, the Holter monitor ECG and possibly electrophysiologic studies will be valuable to obtain more detailed information regarding the patient's arrhythmia. The exact cause of this advanced A-V block is uncertain in this patient, although previous viral infection or cardiac trauma may be considered. In most cases congenital A-V block represents *complete* A-V block and not partial A-V block.

CASE 86

This ECG tracing, obtained from an 80-year-old man, was discussed during a weekly arrhythmia conference. He denied syncope or near syncope, although he had experienced dizziness from time to time. He was *not* taking any medication.

1. What is the cardiac rhythm diagnosis?

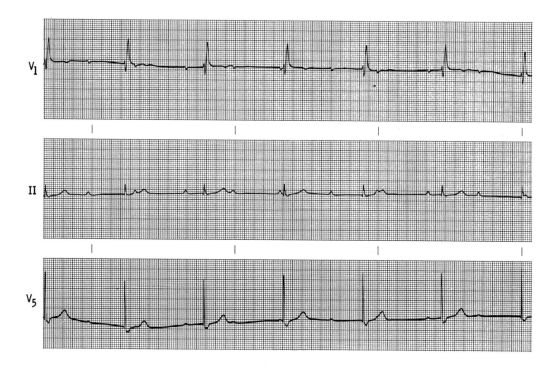

Diagnosis

The cardiac rhythm is sinus (atrial rate: 60 beats per minute), with A-V JER (ventricular rate: 37 beats per minute) due to complete A-V block. Thus there is no relationship between the atrial and ventricular activities, meaning complete A-V dissociation. It should be noted that complete A-V block is one of the commonest underlying cardiac arrhythmias responsible for the production of complete A-V dissociation. The QRS complexes are broad because of RBBB.

A possibility of VER is considered, but it is an unlikely possibility because all QRS complexes exhibit typical RBBB.

This ECG tracing was taken on a 46-year-old man with acute diaphragmatic MI.

1. What is the cardiac rhythm diagnosis?
2. What is the proper therapeutic approach?

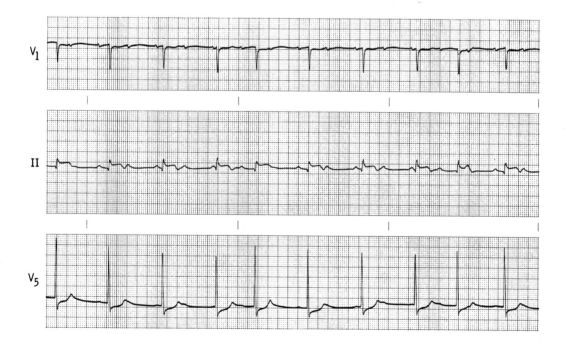

Diagnosis

The cardiac rhythm is sinus tachycardia (atrial rate: 110 beats per minute), with intermittent A-V JER (ventricular rate: 57 beats per minute) due to Wenckebach advanced A-V block, producing incomplete A-V dissociation. Note that there are three conducted sinus beats (the fifth, ninth, and tenth beats).

As described previously, Wenckebach A-V block in acute diaphragmatic MI is a transient phenomenon in most cases (*see* Case 83 which is the same patient), and no active treatment is necessary as long as the A-V block does not produce a significant symptom or hemodynamic abnormality. By and large the patient remains asymptomatic as long as the ventricular rate is not too slow (around 40–60 beats per minute).

LVH is considered (*see* Case 10).

DI was suspected in a 56-year-old woman
with chronic CHF.

1. What is the cardiac rhythm diagnosis?

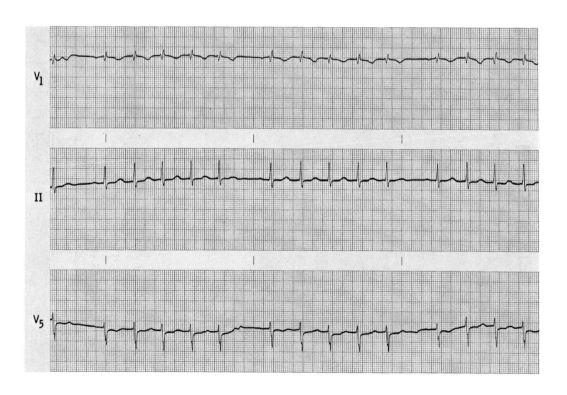

Diagnosis

The cardiac rhythm is sinus tachycardia (atrial rate: 108 beats per minute), with 6 : 5 Wenckebach A-V block. Note that the PR intervals progressively lengthen, and the RR intervals simultaneously, progressively shorten until a blocked P wave occurs. In general, Wenckebach conduction must always be considered whenever there are grouped beats followed by a ventricular pause. Inexperienced readers may have some difficulty in recognizing P waves because some waves are superimposed on the T waves of the preceding beat so that the P waves become less obvious.

In mild cases of DI discontinuation of digitalis alone is often sufficient to restore normal sinus rhythm.

There is incomplete RBBB.

A 77-year-old man was admitted to the intermediate CCU because of a very slow heart rate associated with a near syncope. He was *not* taking any medication.

1. What is the cardiac rhythm diagnosis?

2. What is most likely the underlying disorder?

3. What is the proper therapeutic approach?

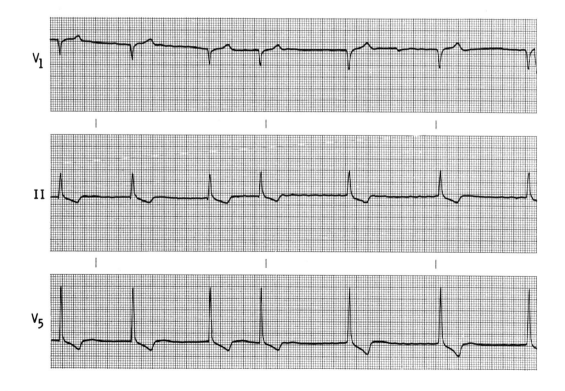

Diagnosis

The cardiac rhythm is AF, with advanced A-V block producing very slow ventricular rate (rate: 38–45 beats per minute) and intermittent A-V JEBs. Note that some RR intervals are regular, with slow ventricular rate meaning intermittent A-V JEBs.

When dealing with AF with a slow ventricular rate with or without A-V JEBs or VEBs, SSS should always be considered as a possible underlying disorder. Of course the above-mentioned arrhythmia should *not* be drug-induced rhythm disorder.

Various ECG manifestations of SSS are summarized as follows:

ECG Manifestations of SSS

1. Marked and persisting sinus bradycardia.
2. Sinus arrest and/or SA block.
3. Drug (eg, atropine, Isuprel)-resistant sinus bradyarrhythmias.
4. Long pause following an APC.
5. Prolonged sinus node recovery time determined by atrial pacing.
6. Chronic AF or repetitive occurrence of AF (less commonly atrial flutter): (a) with slow ventricular rate; and (b) preceded or followed by sinus bradycardia, sinus arrest, or S-A block.
7. A-V JER (chronic).
8. Carotid sinus syncope.
9. Failure of restoration of sinus rhythm following cardioversion.
10. BTS.
11. Common coexisting A-V block and/or intraventricular block.
12. Any combination of the above.

Permanent artificial pacing is considered to be indicated for symptomatic and/or advanced SSS.

Diagnosis of LVH is made using the conventional criteria (*see* Case 10).

This ECG tracing was recorded from a 75-year-old woman who was admitted to the CCU because of a recent heart attack.

1. What is the cardiac rhythm diagnosis?

2. What is the ECG diagnosis?
3. What is the proper therapeutic approach to this arrhythmia?

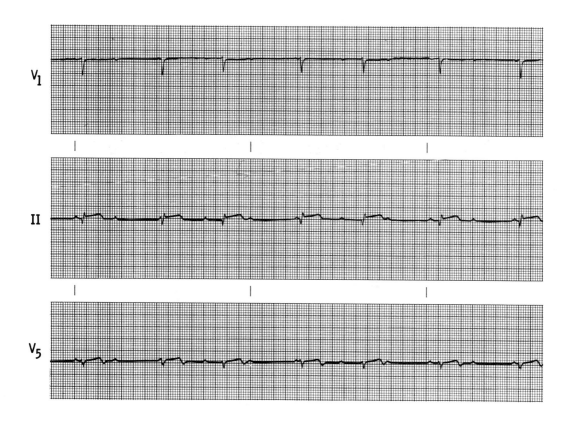

Diagnosis

The cardiac rhythm is sinus (atrial rate: 78 beats per minute), with advanced Wenckebach A-V block causing intermittent A-V JEBs (ventricular rate: 46 beats per minute). Thus there is incomplete A-V dissociation. There are three conducted sinus beats (the third, fifth, and sixth beats), and the remaining QRS complexes represent A-V JEBs.

The diagnosis of diaphragmatic-lateral MI can be made using the conventional criteria (only leads V_1, II, and V_5 are shown here).

As stressed earlier, no active treatment is necessary for Wenckebach A-V block associated with acute diaphragmatic MI as long as the arrhythmia causes no significant symptom or hemodynamic abnormality (see Cases 83 and 87).

This ECG tracing, which belongs to a 54-year-old female, was discussed during a weekly advanced arrhythmia conference. She was *not* taking any medication but had experienced several episodes of near syncope.

1. What is the cardiac rhythm diagnosis?
2. What is the proper way of handling her arrhythmia?

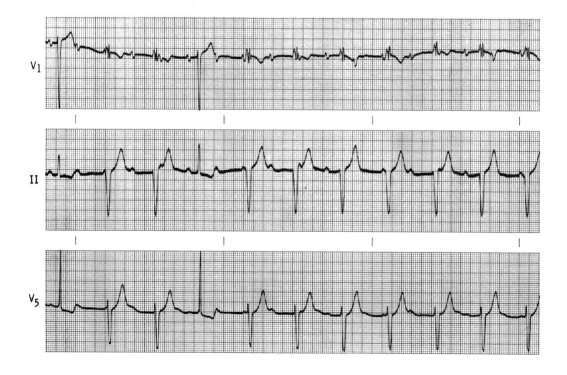

Diagnosis

The cardiac rhythm is sinus tachycardia (atrial rate: 110 beats per minute), with advanced A-V block and intermittent nonparoxysmal VT (accelerated idioventricular rhythm or idioventricular tachycardia, rate: 64 beats per minute), producing incomplete A-V dissociation. The type of A-V block *cannot* be determined with certainty, but it is most likely Mobitz type II A-V block because accelerated VER (idioventricular tachycardia) occurs as a result of A-V block. Remember that advanced Wenckebach A-V block usually produces A-V JER because the block is within the A-V junction (A-V nodal block). On the other hand, Mobitz type II A-V block represents infranodal block. There are two conducted sinus beats (the first and fourth beats).

Holter monitor ECG and EPS are highly recommended in this patient to obtain detailed information regarding her arrhythmia. Permanent artificial pacing is most likely indicated because Mobitz type II A-V block is irreversible in most cases, and the arrhythmia is symptomatic in this case.

LVH is diagnosed, and LAH is considered (*see* Cases 10 and 33).

CASE 92

A 79-year-old hypertensive woman was examined at the cardiac clinic during a periodic medical checkup. She has been taking hydrochlorothiazide, 50 mg, every other day.

1. What is the cardiac arrhythmia?
2. What is the ECG diagnosis?

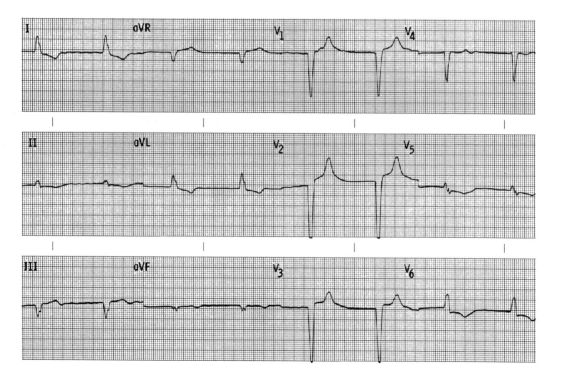

Diagnosis

The cardiac rhythm is AF, with A-V JER (rate: 44 beats per minute) due to complete A-V block. Thus there is complete A-V dissociation. The RR intervals are regular throughout, and the atrial and ventricular activities are independent.

The diagnosis of LBBB is made using the conventional criteria (see Case 33). In addition, diaphragmatic MI is considered.

CASE 93

This ECG tracing, obtained from a 71-year-old woman, was discussed during a weekly ECG conference.

1. What is the cardiac rhythm diagnosis?

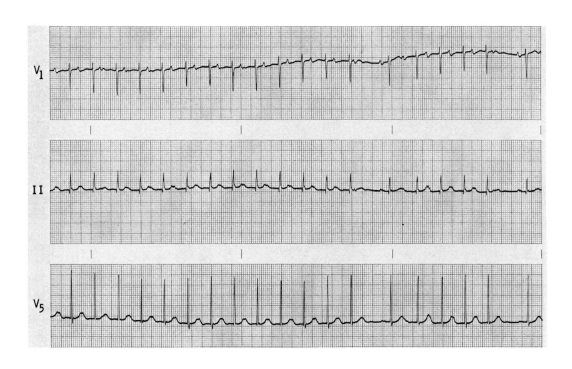

Diagnosis

The cardiac rhythm is sinus tachycardia (atrial rate: 130 beats per minute), with very slowly progressing Wenckebach A-V block (see Case 82) and two blocked APCs or reciprocal beats. The usual Wenckebach A-V block is interrupted by a blocked APC or a reciprocal beat. Note that a blocked premature P wave is observed during a ventricular pause.

Many inexperienced readers may *not* recognize sinus P waves because they are superimposed on the T waves of the preceding beats in most areas. In addition, some readers may misinterpret the premature ectopic P wave, which is blocked.

DI was considered to be the underlying disorder that produced the patient's arrhythmia.

CASE 94

Cardiac consultation was requested on a 63-year-old woman with chronic renal failure.

1. What is the cardiac rhythm diagnosis?
2. What is the ECG diagnosis?

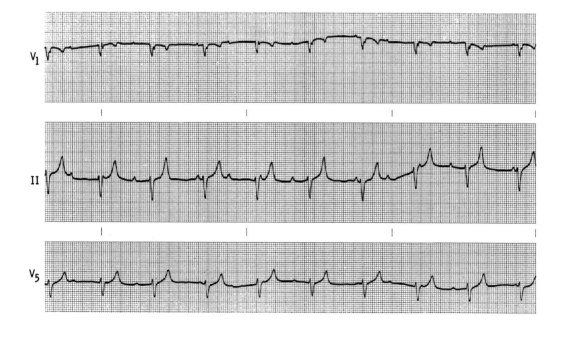

Diagnosis

Cardiac rhythm is sinus (atrial rate: 92 beats per minute), with A-V JER (ventricular rate: 55 beats per minute) due to complete A-V block. Thus there is complete A-V dissociation.

It should be noted that the T waves are peaked and tall in leads II and V$_5$, and the QRS complexes are slightly widened, with left axis deviation indicative of left anterior hemiblock (*see* Case 27). These ECG changes are considered to be due to hyperkalemia.

Various ECG manifestations of hyperkalemia are summarized as follows:

ECG Manifestations of Hyperkalemia

- Tent-shaped and tall T waves with narrow base (mild cases).
- Flattening of P waves (mild to moderately advanced cases).
- Varying degree A-V block (moderately advanced cases).
- Various intraventricular blocks (moderately advanced cases).
- VPCs followed by VT and fibrillation (advanced cases).
- Ventricular standstill (far-advanced cases).

This ECG tracing was taken on a 79-year-old woman with chronic AF. DI was suspected when she developed a slow and regular rhythm.

1. What is the cardiac rhythm diagnosis?

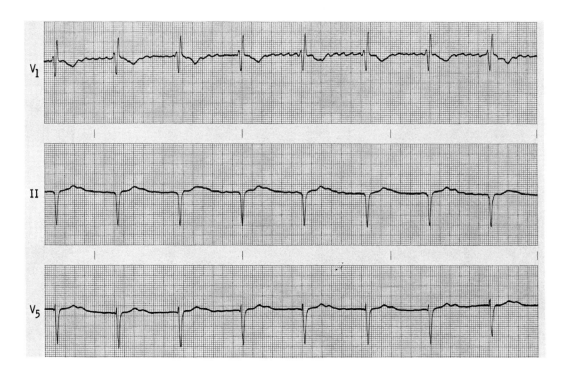

Diagnosis

The cardiac rhythm is atrial flutter-fibrillation, with A-V JER (ventricular rate: 48 beats per minute) due to complete A-V block. Thus there is complete A-V dissociation.

The diagnosis of RBBB can be made using conventional criteria (*see* Case 34). In addition, marked left axis deviation of the QRS complexes (the axis estimated to be −75 degrees is indicative of left anterior hemiblock. Therefore the diagnosis of BFB is established (*see* Case 7).

A possibility of diaphragmatic-lateral MI is raised in view of QS waves in leads II, III, and aVF and markedly reduced R wave amplitude with Q waves in leads V_{4-6} (only leads II and V_5 are shown here).

Prominent U waves are suggestive of hypokalemia, which frequently predisposes to DI.

This ECG tracing, which belongs to a 62-year-old female, was discussed during a weekly arrhythmia conference. She was *not* taking any drug and denied any syncopal episode.

1. What is the cardiac rhythm diagnosis?

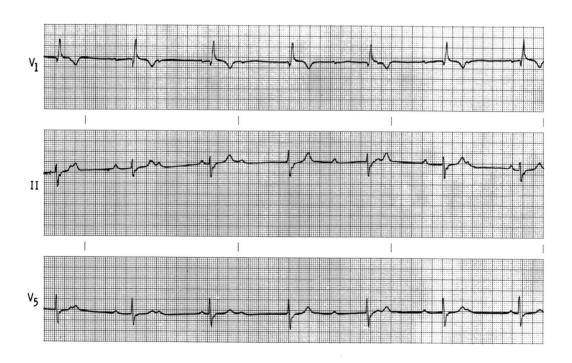

Diagnosis

The cardiac rhythm is sinus (atrial rate: 72 beats per minute), with A-V JER (ventricular rate: 40 beats per minute) due to complete A-V block. Therefore there is complete A-V dissociation.

The diagnosis of BFB consisting of RBBB and left anterior hemiblock can be established using the conventional criteria (*see* Case 7).

The escape rhythm may be arising from the posterior fascicle of the left bundle branch system judging from the configuration of the QRS complexes (RBBB with left anterior hemiblock pattern).

The Holter monitor ECG and EPS should be considered seriously to obtain detailed information regarding the characteristics of this patient's A-V block. When the A-V block is determined to be infranodal block, permanent pacing is definitely indicated.

CASE 97

A 59-year-old woman with a history of a previous heart attack was admitted to intermediate CCU because she developed a new cardiac arrhythmia, which was considered to be due to DI.

1. What is the cardiac rhythm diagnosis?
2. What is the proper way to handle her arrhythmia?

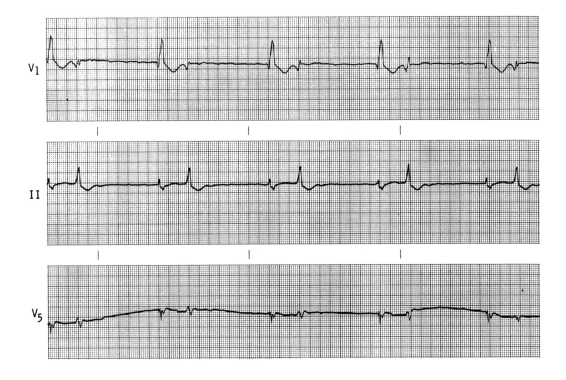

V₁

II

V₅

Diagnosis

The cardiac rhythm is AF, with A-V JER (ventricular rate: 55 beats per minute) due to complete A-V block and frequent VPCs producing ventricular bigeminy. When dealing with the above-mentioned cardiac arrhythmia, the diagnosis of advanced DI is almost certain.

The diagnosis of RBBB can be made using the conventional criteria (*see* Case 34). The patient's 12-lead ECG shows old extensive anterior MI (only leads V_1, II, and V_5 are shown here).

A temporary artificial pacing should be considered if her arrhythmia produces any significant symptom or hemodynamic abnormality. Otherwise discontinuation of digitalis may be sufficient to restore her original basic cardiac rhythm. Potassium administration is definitely beneficial if the serum potassium level is found to be low. Phenytoin (Dilantin) is effective to suppress ventricular arrhythmia induced by digitalis.

These two ECG tracings were obtained from a 46-year-old man with acute heart attack. Tracing **A** represents his cardiac rhythm strips, whereas tracing **B** is his 12-lead ECG.

1. What is the cardiac rhythm diagnosis?
2. What is the proper therapeutic approach?

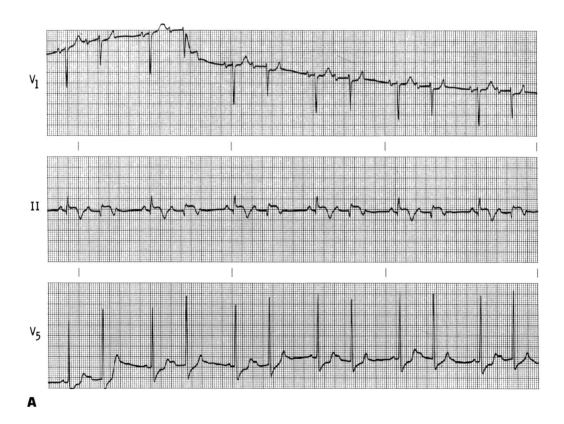

A

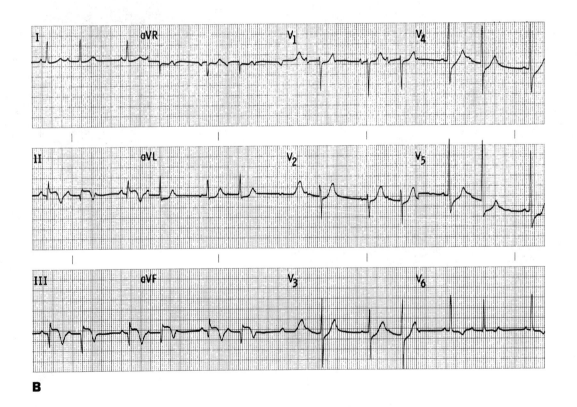

B

4. ATRIOVENTRICULAR BLOCK: Case 98

Diagnosis

The cardiac rhythm is sinus tachycardia (atrial rate: 115 beats per minute), with 3 : 2 Wenckebach A-V block (ventricular rate: 76 beats per minute). The other QRS complexes are slightly deformed because of aberrant ventricular conduction. Aberrant ventricular conduction occurs as a result of Ashman's phenomenon, which is explained in detail below. This is the same patient as Cases 83 and 87.

Ashman's Phenomenon

The most important factor for the production of aberrant ventricular conduction is Ashman's phenomenon. In 1945 Ashman had described the ECG finding that aberrant ventricular conduction tends to occur following a long ventricular cycle (RR interval) preceding the coupling interval (the interval from a bizarre beat to the normal beat of the basic rhythm). It can be said that the longer the ventricular cycle (RR interval) the longer the refractory period following it; the shorter the ventricular cycle the shorter the refractory period.

Diagnostic Criteria of Ashman's Phenomenon

1. Ashman's phenomenon may be recognized in any cardiac rhythm when aberrant ventricular conduction occurs following a long ventricular cycle (RR interval).
2. The aberrant ventricular conduction is more pronounced in a ventricular complex following the longest ventricular cycle as a result of marked Ashman's phenomenon.
3. Atrial or A-V junctional bigeminy nearly always shows aberrant ventricular conduction in atrial or A-V

junctional premature beats because of Ashman's phenomenon. This is observed because atrial of A-V junctional premature beats must follow a long ventricular cycle (postectopic pause) during atrial of A-V junctional bigeminy. The same principle can be applied to any form of bigeminal rhythm such as 3 : 2 Wenckebach A-V block.
4. The PR interval of an atrial or A-V junctional premature beat is often long during bigeminy, again as a result of Ashman's phenomenon. For the same reason blocked APCs are common during atrial bigeminy (blocked atrial bigeminy).
5. Ashman's phenomenon is pronounced when the ventricular cycle becomes suddenly shortened following a long ventricular cycle, particularly in AF. As a result aberrant ventricular conduction occurs. It is common to observe consecutively occurring aberrant ventricular conduction once it is initiated by Ashman's phenomenon. This ECG finding closely simulates VT.
6. Ashman's phenomenon may be encountered in MAT, which leads to aberrant ventricular conduction.
7. Occasionally a sinus beat (ventricular captured beat) during incomplete A-V dissociation may show aberrant ventricular conduction as a result of Ashman's phenomenon.
8. The configuration of the QRS complex during aberrant ventricular conduction as a result of Ashman's phenomenon is commonly that of a

RBBB pattern, about 80–85 percent of cases, and only 15–20 percent may show LBBB pattern. Not uncommonly, aberrantly conducted beats may reveal an ECG finding of BFB pattern consisting of RBBB pattern and left anterior or posterior hemiblock pattern. At times aberrantly conducted beats may show both LBBB pattern and RBBB pattern in the same ECG tracing. The alteration of the QRS contour in aberrant ventricular conduction represents functional (not true) bundle branch block and/or hemiblock.

9. The secondary T wave change is observed in an aberrantly conducted QRS complex. The T wave alteration in this circumstance is analogous to that of VPCs or LBBB or RBBB.

The diagnosis of acute diaphragmatic MI is obvious, and also there is LVH.

No active treatment is necessary for this patient's arrhythmia because Wenckebach A-V block associated with acute diaphragmatic MI is a transient phenomenon and is self-limited in almost all cases.

CHAPTER FIVE

SINUS ARRHYTHMIAS

This ECG tracing was taken on a healthy 26-year-old woman.

1. What is the cardiac rhythm diagnosis?

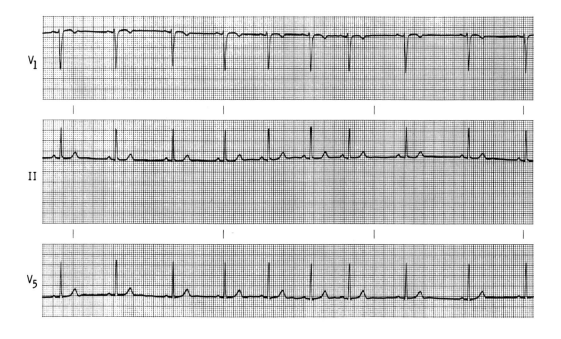

Diagnosis

The cardiac rhythm is sinus arrhythmia, with rates ranging from 50–73 beats per minute. Thus in some areas there is sinus bradycardia. Sinus arrhythmia often coexists with sinus bradycardia.

The diagnosis of sinus arrhythmia is entertained when the variations of the sinus PP cycles are 0.16 second or greater.

Sinus arrhythmia is classified into two major categories—respiratory and nonrespiratory. *Respiratory sinus arrhythmia* is almost a rule rather than an exception in children and young adults. The PP cycles vary according to the respiratory cycles in respiratory sinus arrhythmia. On the other hand, in *nonrespiratory sinus arrhythmia* the PP cycles vary independent of the respiratory cycles. Nonrespiratory sinus arrhythmia is usually found in elderly people or cardiac patients, and other names such as idiopathic sinus arrhythmia have been used. In some cases marked sinus arrhythmia may be an early sign of SSS (*see* Case 89).

CASE 100

This ECG tracing, which belongs to a 72-year-old man, was discussed during a weekly student ECG conference in the evaluation of the P wave configurations. The patient was found to be mildly hypertensive.

1. What is the cardiac rhythm diagnosis?

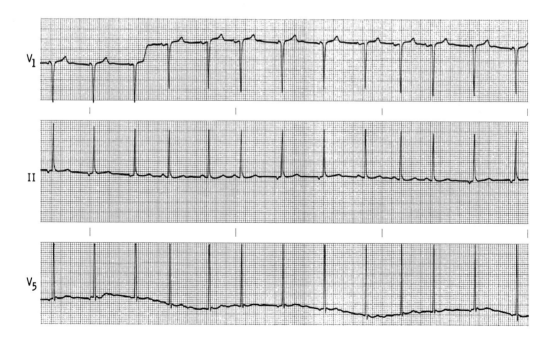

Diagnosis

The cardiac rhythm is sinus arrhythmia, with wandering atrial pacemaker. Note that the PP cycles vary, and also the P wave configurations vary.

Since wandering atrial pacemaker almost always coexists with sinus arrhythmia, many authors consider wandering atrial pacemaker to be an exaggerated form of sinus arrhythmia.

The diagnosis of LVH is established using the conventional criteria (*see* Case 10).

A 79-year-old man was admitted to the CCU for the evaluation of several episodes of syncope or near syncope associated with severe chest pain. He was *not* taking any medication.

1. What is the cardiac rhythm diagnosis?
2. What is the proper therapeutic approach to his arrhythmia?
3. What is the ECG diagnosis?

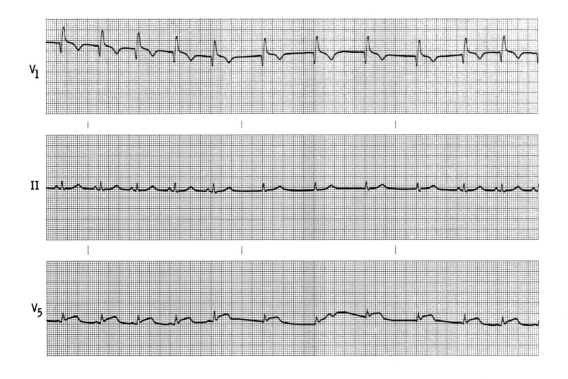

Diagnosis

The basic cardiac rhythm is sinus (rate: 82 beats per minute), but no P wave is discernible in a midportion of the tracing. The absent P waves indicate a period of sinus arrest, meaning that the sinus node fails to produce any cardiac impulse. During sinus arrest there is intermittent A-V JER (the sixth, seventh, eighth, and ninth beats) with a rate of 60 beats per minute.

Sinus arrest is a relatively common sign of SSS, especially in elderly people.

The diagnosis of acute extensive anterior MI (QS or Q wave in all precordial leads in 12-lead ECG) associated with RBBB can be made (see Case 34) using the conventional diagnostic criteria.

Permanent artificial pacing should strongly be considered for symptomatic and/or advanced SSS. However, RBBB itself is rather an insignificant finding even in the presence of acute, extensive, anterior MI.

CASE 102

This ECG tracing, obtained from a 59-year-old man with long-standing hypertension, was discussed during a weekly arrhythmia conference.

1. What is the cardiac rhythm diagnosis?

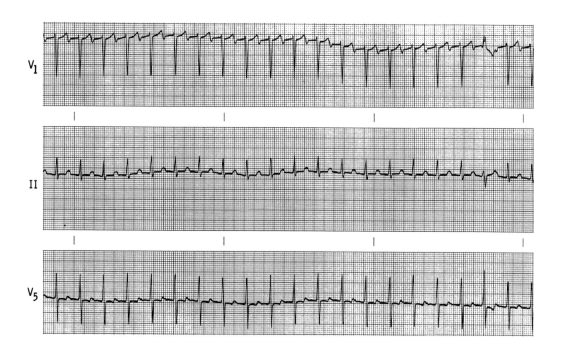

V₁

II

V₅

Diagnosis

The cardiac rhythm is sinus tachycardia (rate: 128 beats per minute), with first degree A-V block. Some inexperienced readers may *not* recognize P waves because they are superimposed on the T waves of the preceding beats. Note a VPC (the second beat from the last).

The diagnosis of LAH as well as LVH is strongly considered (*see* Cases 10 and 33).

CASE 103

These ECG rhythm strips were recorded from a 65-year-old man with many episodes of syncope. He was *not* taking any drug.

1. What is the cardiac rhythm diagnosis?
2. What is the best therapeutic approach?

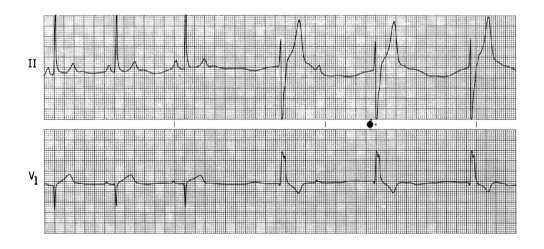

Diagnosis

The underlying cardiac rhythm is sinus bradycardia (rate: 47 beats per minute), but sinus arrest occurs after three sinus beats. Note a blocked P wave in the midportion of the tracing. During sinus arrest VER (rate: 32 beats per minute) is present (the last three beats).

The above-mentioned ECG findings represent manifestations of advanced SSS. Diseased A-V node is strongly considered because the expected A-V JER fails to occur so that VER is produced instead. It has been shown that diseased A-V node is common in SSS.

Permanent artificial pacing is urgently needed for symptomatic advanced SSS.

This ECG tracing, which was taken on an 81-year-old man, was discussed during a weekly advanced arrhythmia conference, with particular emphasis placed on the variations of the PP cycles. He was *not* taking any drug but had several episodes of near syncope.

1. What is the cardiac rhythm diagnosis?
2. What is most likely the underlying disorder?

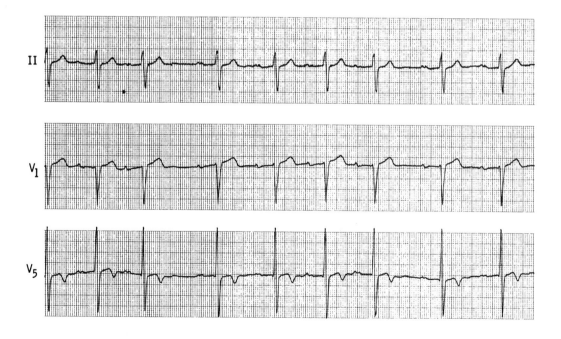

Diagnosis

The basic rhythm is sinus, with first-degree–A-V block (rate: 55 beats per minute), but the PP cycles vary, namely, the PP intervals progressively shorten until a pause occurs. This ECG finding is a characteristic feature of Wenckebach S-A block. The conduction ratio is 5:4. Thus complete cardiac rhythm diagnosis is sinus rhythm, with first degree A-V block and 5:4 Wenckebach S-A block.

If any reader has difficulty in understanding Wenckebach S-A block, he or she should study Wenckebach A-V block in depth (see Case 82).

S-A block is one of the common manifestations of SSS (see Case 89). S-A block not uncommonly coexists with A-V block, as seen in this case.

There are various other ECG abnormalities in this tracing, including left anterior hemiblock, LAH, and LVH (see Cases 10, 27, and 33).

CASE 105

A permanent artificial pacemaker was implanted on an 84-year-old woman 6 months earlier because of syncopal episodes.

1. What is the cardiac rhythm diagnosis?
2. What is the underlying disorder that required artificial pacing?

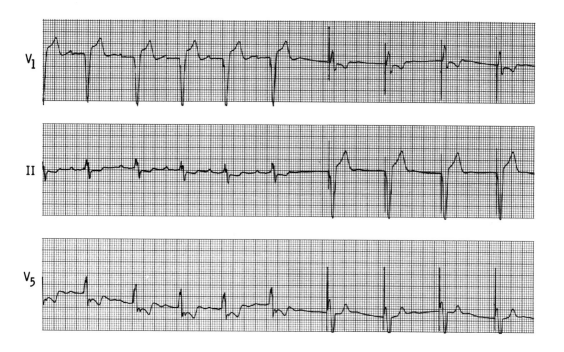

Diagnosis

The cardiac rhythm is sinus, with first-degree–A-V block (rate: 73 beats per minute) and intermittent sinus arrest. During sinus arrest demand ventricular pacemaker rhythm takes over the ventricular activity (ventricular rate: 60 beats per minute).

The diagnosis of LBBB can be made using the conventional criteria (*see* Case 33).

Malposition of the pacemaker electrode is considered because the QRS complex in lead V_1 shows RS pattern. Remember that lead V_1 should reveal QS complex when the pacemaker electrode is in the right ventricular apex (correct position).

The patient's underlying disorder is advanced SSS, which is manifested by sinus arrest, which requires permanent artificial pacing (*see* Case 89).

CASE 106

This Holter monitor ECG was obtained from an 80-year-old woman with syncope episodes. She was not taking any drugs when the Holter monitor ECG was recorded. Her 12-lead ECG showed sinus bradycardia (rate: 55 beats per minute) with occasional VPCs and a nonspecific abnormality of the T waves (not shown here).

1. What is the cardiac rhythm diagnosis?
2. What is the treatment of choice?

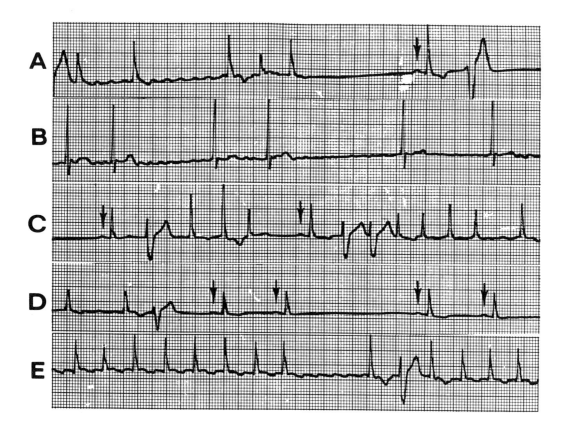

Diagnosis

The cardiac rhythm strips **A** through **E** are *not* continuous. Note the sinus P waves (arrows). The cardiac rhythm is a very unstable and slow sinus bradycardia, with periods of sinus arrest, a paroxysmal AF, advanced A-V block, and a paroxysmal atrial flutter. In addition there are many bizarre QRS complexes; the majority of them are due to aberrant ventricular conduction, but some of them are VPCs.

The cardiac rhythm on this Holter monitor ECG is a typical example of a BTS due to a far-advanced SSS. The treatment of choice is, again, implantation of a permanent artificial pacemaker. In addition, one or more antiarrhythmic drugs may be needed when the tachyarrhythmia component persists after pacing. SSS has been discussed in detail elsewhere (*see* Case 89).

CHAPTER SIX

ATRIAL ARRHYTHMIAS

CASE 107

This ECG tracing was taken on a 65-year-old woman as part of her annual medical checkup. She had no complaint.

1. What is the cardiac rhythm diagnosis?
2. What is the proper therapeutic approach?

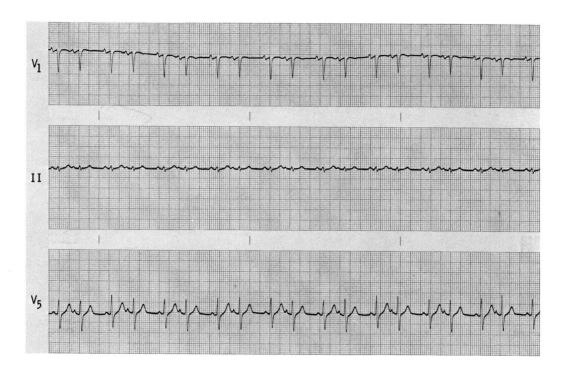

Diagnosis

The basic cardiac rhythm is sinus tachycardia, with a rate of 114 beats per minute. There are frequent APCs, producing atrial bigeminy. Note that all QRS complexes of APCs are slightly deformed (more pronounced in lead V_1) due to minimum aberrant ventricular conduction as a result of Ashman's phenomenon (see Case 98).

By and large no active treatment is necessary for APCs as long as the patient does not experience any symptom (eg, palpitation). However, any unusual personal habits (eg, excessive consumption of coffee) should be avoided if the APCs are considered to be due to the above-mentioned reasons. A variety of arrhythmias, including APCs, are commonly encountered in patients with MVPS and hyperthyroidism. These facts should be kept in mind whenever dealing with unexplainable cardiac arrhythmias.

Cardiac consultation was requested on a 63-year-old woman with mild COPD for the evaluation of her cardiac arrhythmia.

1. What is the cardiac rhythm diagnosis?
2. What is the proper therapeutic approach?

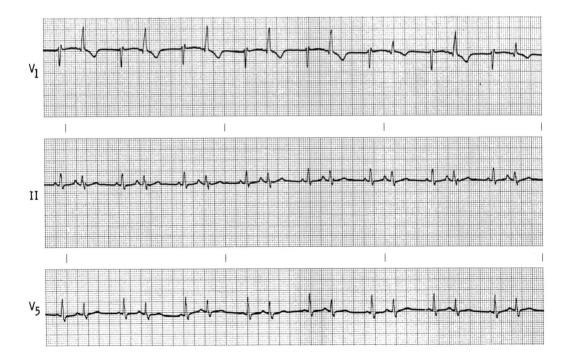

Diagnosis

The underlying cardiac rhythm is sinus, with a rate of 100 beats per minute. There are frequent APCs, producing atrial bigeminy. It should be noted that all APCs reveal marked aberrant ventricular conduction as a result of Ashman's phenomenon (*see* Case 98). APCs with aberrant ventricular conduction may easily be misdiagnosed as VPCs when a reader fails to recognize a premature P wave that precedes each bizarre QRS complex.

The basic QRS complexes of the sinus beats show incomplete RBBB.

It is a well-known fact that various atrial arrhythmias, including APCs, are very common in patients with COPD. These atrial arrhythmias are often abolished when the underlying pulmonary disease is well treated.

A 58-year-old man was admitted to the CCU because of acute MI.

1. What is the cardiac rhythm diagnosis?

2. What is the ECG diagnosis?
3. What is the proper way to handle this arrhythmia?

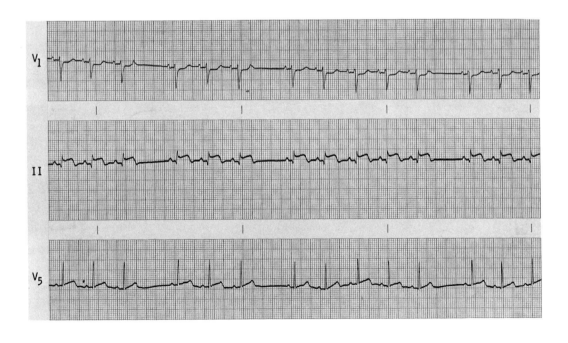

Diagnosis

The underlying rhythm is sinus, with a rate of 94 beats per minute. There are three APCs that are *not* followed by QRS complexes. This finding is called "blocked" (nonconducted) APCs. The blocked APCs are best shown in lead V_1.

Blocked APCs superficially resemble sinus arrhythmia, sinus arrest, and S-A block.

No treatment is necessary for blocked APCs.

The diagnosis of acute diaphragmatic (inferior) MI is obvious on the basis of pathologic Q waves in leads II, III, and aVF (only lead II is shown here), with ST segment elevation and T wave inversion. In addition, posterior subepicardial injury is strongly considered on the basis of ST segment depression in leads V_{1-3} (only lead V_1 is shown here).

CASE 110

A 62-year-old woman was seen in the ER because of a very rapid heart action. She was *not* taking any medication.

1. What is the cardiac rhythm diagnosis?
2. What is the proper way to handle this patient?

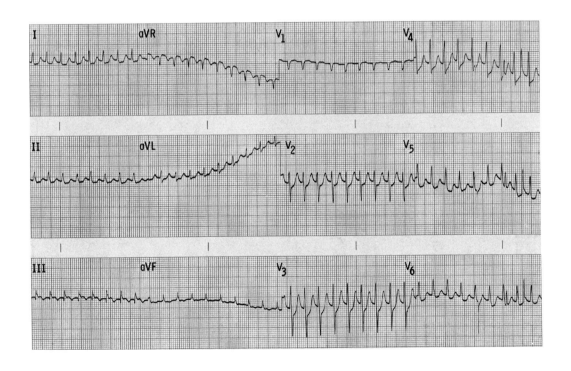

Diagnosis

The cardiac rhythm is regular, and the QRS complexes are normal. No P waves are discernible. Thus the term "supraventricular tachycardia" is applied under this circumstance (the rate: 220 beats per minute). Although the precise diagnosis of this arrhythmia is *not* possible, supraventricular tachycardia usually represents paroxysmal atrial tachycardia, A-V JT, or reciprocating tachycardia.

The first therapeutic approach is the application of CSS. CSS is often effective in terminating supraventricular tachycardia. If CSS is found to be ineffective, various drugs (eg, beta blockers, calcium blockers, digoxin) should be considered. When the clinical situation seems to be urgent (eg, hypotension), DC shock should be applied immediately. EPS is considered only when the arrhythmia is found to be resistant to the conventional drug therapy.

Whenever possible the underlying cause or disorder responsible for the production of the arrhythmia should be investigated and treated as needed. Common underlying causes or disorders include extreme stress, excessive coffee, WPW syndrome (*see* Chapter 9), hyperthyroidism, MVPS, and pulmonary embolism.

An 83-year-old woman was admitted to the intermediate CCU because of rapid heart action. She was *not* taking any medication.

1. What is the cardiac rhythm diagnosis?
2. What is the proper therapeutic approach?

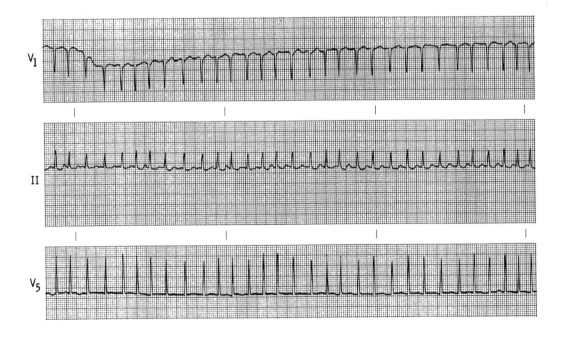

Diagnosis

The cardiac rhythm is AF, with very rapid ventricular response (ventricular rate: 180–220 beats per minute). The ventricular cycle is grossly irregular, with no discernible P waves.

The drug of choice for AF with rapid ventricular response is rapid digitalization. If the clinical situation is urgent, DC shock should be applied immediately.

These cardiac rhythm strips were discussed during a weekly ECG conference primarily in the evaluation of bizarre QRS complexes. These strips were obtained from a 59-year-old man.

1. What is the cardiac rhythm diagnosis?
2. What are the five causes of broad QRS complexes?

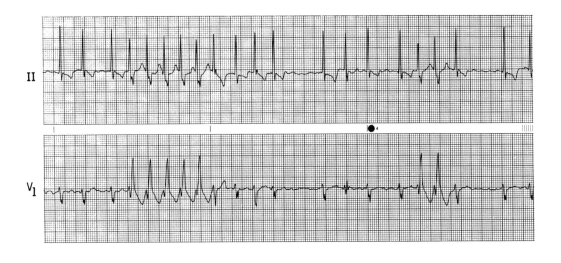

II

V₁

Diagnosis

The cardiac rhythm is AF, with rapid ventricular response (ventricular rate: 130–200 beats per minute). There are many bizarre QRS complexes that represent aberrant ventricular conduction initiated by Ashman's phenomenon (*see* Case 98). The aberrantly conducted beats closely simulate VPCs or a short run of VT. VPCs and VT are excluded on the basis of a lack of any postectopic pause. It should be remembered that a VPC or a short run of VT is always followed by a significant postectopic pause (*see* Chapter 8).

There are five causes of broad (bizarre) QRS complexes as follows:

ECG Findings Causing Broad (Bizarre) QRS Complexes

Ventricular Ectopy

- VPCs.
- Ventricular parasystole.
- VT.
- VEBs or VER.
- VF.

Intraventricular Block

- RBBB.
- LBBB.
- BFB or TFB.
- Diffuse (nonspecific) intraventricular block.

Aberrant Ventricular Conduction

- Ashman's phenomenon.
- Short coupling interval.
- Very rapid supraventricular tachyarrhythmias of various origins or mechanisms.

WPW Syndrome

Artificial Pacemaker-Induced Ventricular Beats or Rhythm

There are three causes of aberrant ventricular conduction, as follows:

1. Ashman's phenomenon.
2. Short coupling interval.
3. Very rapid ventricular rate (usually faster than 180 beats per minute).

A 66-year-old woman developed palpitations suddenly. She was *not* taking any drug.

1. What is the cardiac rhythm diagnosis?
2. What is the proper therapeutic approach?

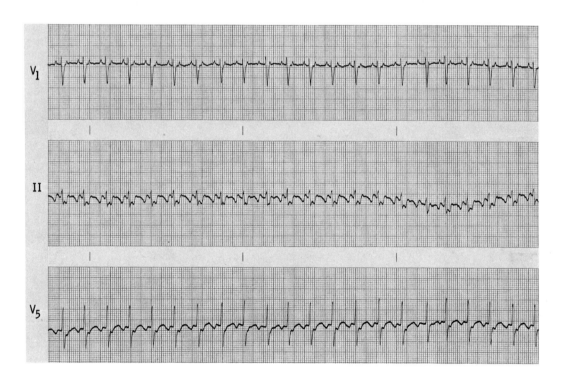

Diagnosis

The cardiac rhythm is atrial flutter (atrial rate: 264 beats per minute), with predominantly 2 : 1 A-V response (ventricular rate: 132 beats per minute).

The therapeutic approach to atrial flutter is very similar to that of AF (*see* Cases 9 and 20). Rapid digitalization is the most effective way to treat atrial flutter with 2 : 1 A-V response.

CASE 114

This ECG tracing, obtained from a 76-year-old woman, was discussed during a weekly arrhythmia conference. She was taking a cardiac drug.

1. What is the cardiac rhythm diagnosis?
2. What cardiac drug most likely was taken by this patient?

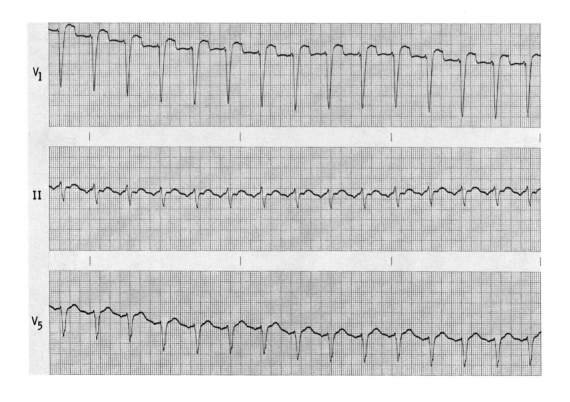

Diagnosis

The cardiac rhythm is atrial flutter (atrial rate: 180 beats per minute), with 2 : 1 A-V response (ventricular rate: 90 beats per minute). The atrial flutter cycle is much slower than usual (the usual atrial flutter cycles range from 250–350 beats per minute) because of quinidine effect.

It has been shown that quinidine or quinidine-like antiarrhythmic agents (eg, procainamide) produce reduction of atrial flutter rate, whereas digitalis causes acceleration of atrial flutter cycle.

A 72-year-old woman with known COPD was seen at the pulmonary clinic during a periodic medical checkup. This tracing was discussed during a weekly arrhythmia conference.

1. What is the cardiac rhythm diagnosis?
2. What is the proper therapeutic approach?

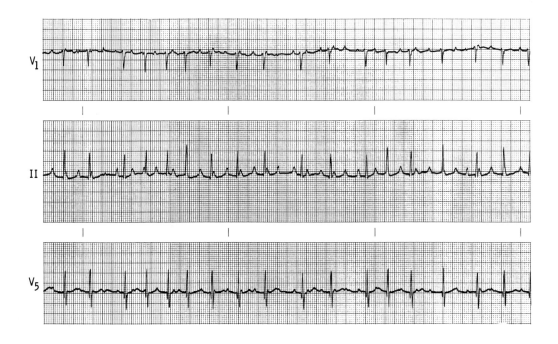

Diagnosis

The cardiac rhythm is MAT, with rates ranging from 180–240 beats per minute. It should be noted that the configurations of the P waves, the PP cycles, and the PR intervals vary throughout the tracing. In addition, many P waves are *not* conducted to the ventricles—also a characteristic feature of MAT. Thus a complete diagnosis of this tracing is MAT with varying A-V block.

Some QRS complexes are slightly deformed because of aberrant ventricular conduction (*see* Case 98).

Clinically MAT is most commonly encountered in patients with COPD. Therefore MAT is best managed when the underlying pulmonary disease is well treated. Various antiarrhythmic agents are often *not* effective for MAT as long as the pulmonary function is *not* improved.

CASE 116

A 72-year-old man was evaluated in a cardiologist's office because he had experienced frequent episodes of dizziness and near syncope. He was *not* taking any drug.

1. What is the cardiac rhythm diagnosis?

2. What is most likely the underlying disorder responsible for the production of his arrhythmia?

3. What is the best therapeutic approach?

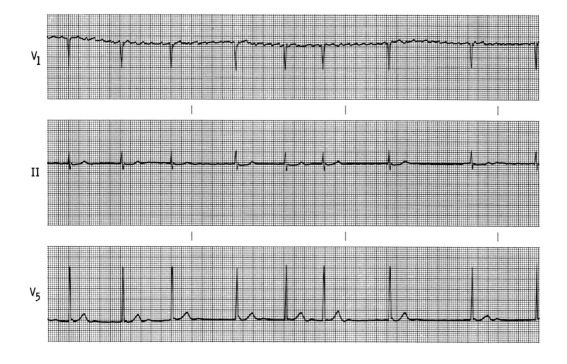

Diagnosis

The cardiac rhythm is AF, with advanced A-V block causing slow ventricular rate (42–55 beats per minute). Some RR intervals are equal (regular) because A-V JEBs occur intermittently as a result of advanced A-V block.

The underlying disorder responsible for the production of this patient's arrhythmia is most likely SSS (*see* Case 89). Artificial pacing is highly recommended for symptomatic and/or advanced SSS.

The diagnosis of LVH is considered by voltage criteria (*see* Case 10).

CASE 117

This is a routine ECG tracing taken on a 68-year-old woman with long-standing hypertension.

1. What is the cardiac rhythm diagnosis?
2. What is the ECG diagnosis?

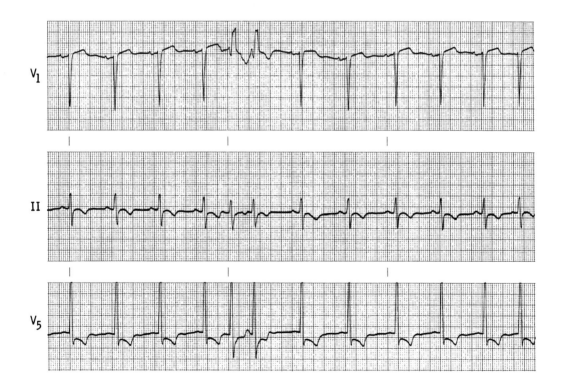

Diagnosis

The underlying cardiac rhythm is sinus
(rate: 68 beats per minute), but there are
frequent APCs. Two APCs occur consecutively (called "atrial group beats") in a
midportion of the tracing (the fifth and
sixth beats), and both APCs show bizarre
QRS complexes because of aberrant ventricular conduction (*see* Case 98).

APCs with aberrant ventricular conduction closely simulate VPCs with group
beats.

The diagnosis of LVH is made using
the conventional criteria (*see* Case 10), and
diffuse myocardial ischemia is also considered (T wave inversion in many leads).

CASE 118

This ECG tracing, which belongs to a 71-year-old woman, was discussed during a weekly student ECG conference.

1. What is the cardiac rhythm diagnosis?

2. What is the ECG diagnosis?
3. What is the best therapeutic approach?

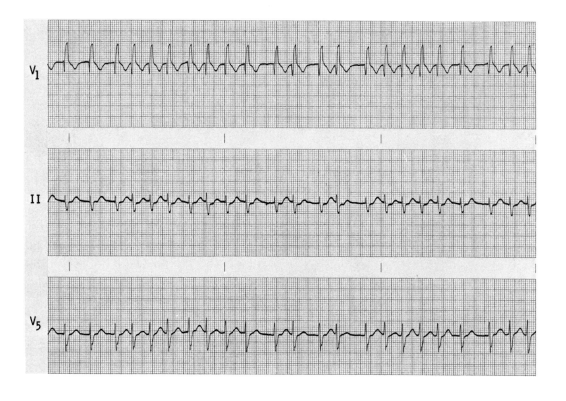

Diagnosis

The cardiac rhythm is AF, with rapid ventricular response (rate: 160–175 beats per minute).

The diagnosis of BFB consisting of RBBB and left anterior hemiblock can be entertained using the conventional criteria (*see* Case 7).

Some inexperienced readers may erroneously diagnose the finding as VT because of broad QRS complexes (RBBB) with rapid ventricular rate (AF). Obviously grossly irregular ventricular cycles with no discernible P waves exclude a possibility of VT.

The drug of choice for AF with rapid ventricular response is rapid digitalization.

This ECG tracing was taken on a 75-year-old man who complained of palpitations. He was not taking any medication.

1. What is the cardiac rhythm diagnosis?
2. What is the ECG diagnosis?

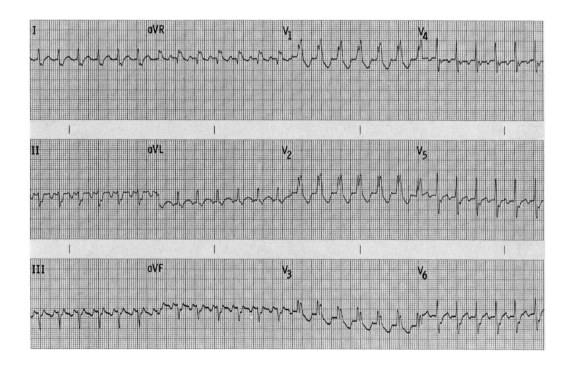

Diagnosis

The cardiac rhythm is atrial flutter (atrial rate: 300 beats per minute), with 2 : 1 A-V conduction (ventricular rate: 150 beats per minute). Some inexperienced readers may misdiagnose the finding as supraventricular tachycardia, AT, A-V JT, and even VT. In some ECG leads atrial flutter waves are not clearly shown because of their superimposition to the end portion of the QRS complexes.

The diagnosis of BFB consisting of RBBB and left anterior hemiblock can be entertained using the conventional diagnostic criteria (see Case 7). As described previously, a combination of RBBB and left anterior hemiblock is the commonest ECG manifestation of incomplete BBBB (see Case 7).

This ECG tracing was obtained from a 69-year-old man with previous history of anteroseptal MI 1 year earlier.

1. What is the cardiac rhythm diagnosis?

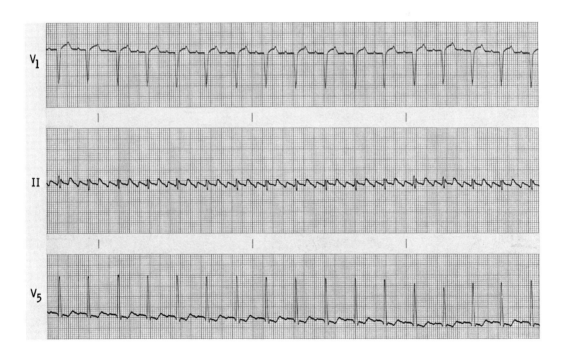

Diagnosis

The cardiac rhythm is atrial flutter (atrial rate: 321 beats per minute), with 3 : 1 A-V block (ventricular rate: 107 beats per minute). The 3 : 1 A-V conduction ratio in atrial flutter is a rather unusual manifestation. A pure form of atrial flutter almost always shows 2 : 1 A-V conduction, and often 4 : 1 A-V block is produced when the A-V conduction is delayed by digitalization or other drugs (eg, beta blockers).

The diagnosis of LVH is considered (*see* Case 10).

CASE 121

These cardiac rhythm strips, taken on a 70-year-old man, were discussed during a weekly arrhythmia conference.

1. What is the cardiac rhythm diagnosis?

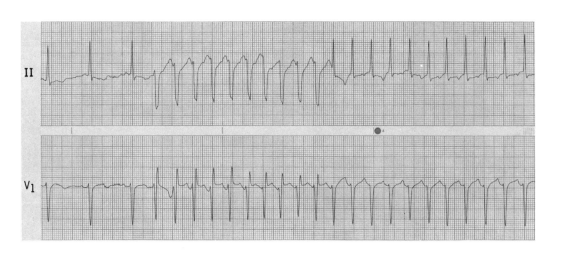

II

V₁

Diagnosis

The underlying cardiac rhythm is sinus (rate: 70 beats per minute), but the cardiac rhythm is changed suddenly after three sinus beats, namely, PAT occurs with rates ranging from 160–175 beats per minute. It is interesting to note that the first half of PAT demonstrates bizarre QRS complexes because of aberrant ventricular conduction (see Case 98).

Under this circumstance aberrant ventricular conduction occurs because the ventricular rate suddenly increases during PAT. Thus the initiation of aberrant ventricular conduction in this case is somewhat comparable to the Ashman's phenomenon (see Case 98).

Needless to say, VT is superficially simulated during PAT with aberrant ventricular conduction (see Case 112).

This ECG tracing was recorded from a 75-year-old man with known COPD.

1. What is the cardiac rhythm diagnosis?

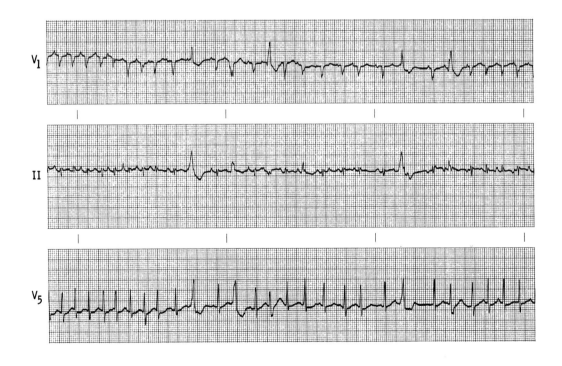

Diagnosis

At a glance the cardiac rhythm appears to be AF because the ventricular cycle is grossly irregular, and the P waves are *not* clearly visible in most areas. However, the correct rhythm diagnosis is MAT. There are many types of P waves, and the PR intervals as well as the PP cycles vary throughout the tracing. These ECG findings are the characteristic features of MAT (*see* Case 115).

There are frequent VPCs, but some bizarre beats represent aberrant ventricular conduction (eg, the last bizarre beat).

As mentioned previously, MAT is most commonly encountered in patients with COPD.

This ECG tracing, which was obtained from a 59-year-old man, was discussed during a weekly ECG conference for the evaluation of bizarre QRS complexes. He was *not* taking any medication.

1. What is the cardiac rhythm diagnosis?

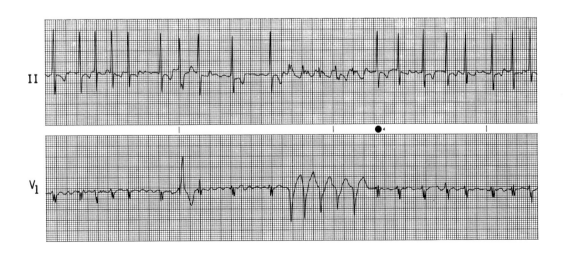

Diagnosis

The cardiac rhythm is AF, with frequent aberrant ventricular conduction. Aberrant ventricular conduction occurs as a result of Ashman's phenomenon (*see* Case 98). Aberrantly conducted beats closely mimic VPCs or a short run of VT.

Various circumstances that cause broad QRS complexes are summarized elsewhere in this book (*see* Case 112). Likewise three causes of aberrant ventricular conduction have been described previously (*see* Case 112).

A 72-year-old man developed a rapid heart action suddenly while this ECG tracing was taken.

1. What is the cardiac rhythm diagnosis?
2. What is the proper way of handling this patient as far as his cardiac arrhythmia is concerned?

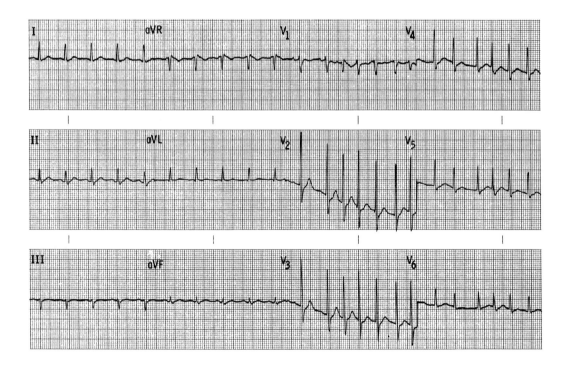

Diagnosis

The underlying cardiac rhythm is sinus tachycardia, with a rate of 110 beats per minute. The cardiac rhythm has changed to paroxysmal AF in the midportion of the ECG tracing.

If this patient develops paroxysmal AF from time to time, the arrhythmia should be prevented, particularly when symptomatic. Slow oral digitalization may be effective to prevent paroxysmal AF. If AF recurs even after digitalization, oral quinidine may be added for the same purpose (0.3–0.4 g four times daily).

A possible underlying cause or disorder responsible for the production of recurrent AF should be investigated. Common causes or underlying disorders may include severe emotional stress; excessive consumption of coffee, alcohol, or cola drinks; cigarette smoking; hyperthyroidism; MVPS; and RHD.

CASE 125

This ECG tracing, taken on a 56-year-old man, was discussed during a weekly advanced arrhythmia conference. He was asymptomatic and was *not* taking any medication.

1. What is the cardiac rhythm diagnosis?
2. What is the proper therapeutic approach?

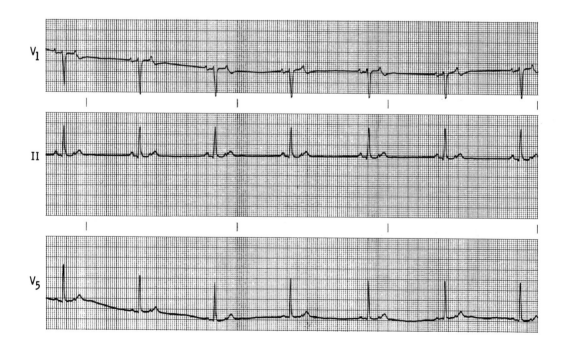

Diagnosis

Many inexperienced readers may simply consider the finding to be marked sinus bradycardia because the ectopic premature P waves may *not* be recognized readily.

The underlying cardiac rhythm is sinus, but there are frequent APCs producing atrial bigeminy. In addition all ectopic P waves are *not* conducted to the ventricles, causing blocked or nonconducted APCs. Thus the correct rhythm diagnosis is frequent blocked APCs causing blocked atrial bigeminy. All ectopic P waves are blocked because the ectopic atrial impulses are conducted during an absolute refractory period in the A-V junction. Very

short coupling intervals and Ashman's phenomenon are responsible for blocked APCs under this circumstance (*see* Case 98). An alternative rhythm diagnosis is blocked reciprocal beats (atrial echo beats).

No active treatment is necessary for APCs, whether conducted or blocked, as long as the patient is asymptomatic from the arrhythmia itself.

Blocked APCs superficially simulate many other arrhythmias, including sinus bradycardia, sinus arrhythmia, sinus arrest, S-A block, and second degree A-V block.

This ECG tracing was taken on a 58-year-old man in the intermediate cardiac care unit. He has been taking digoxin, 0.25 mg, once daily, and quinidine, 0.4 g, four times daily, for several days.

1. What is the cardiac rhythm diagnosis?
2. What is the ECG diagnosis?

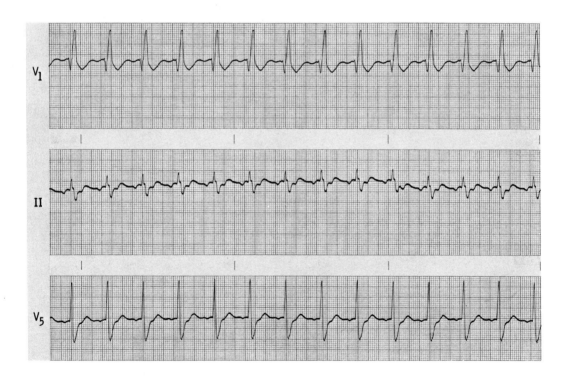

Diagnosis

Some inexperienced readers may misdiagnose the finding as A-V JT or even sinus rhythm. However, the correct rhythm diagnosis is slow atrial flutter (atrial rate: 176 beats per minute), with 2:1 A-V conduction (ventricular rate: 88 beats per minute). Needless to say, the unusually slow atrial flutter cycle is due to quinidine effect.

Before quinidine therapy, this patient's atrial flutter rate was 250 beats per minute. It is important to remember that the atrial flutter cycle is accelerated by digitalis, whereas quinidine produces slowing of the atrial flutter cycle. When digitalis and quinidine are given together, the flutter cycle will be determined by each patient's response to both drugs. Thus the atrial flutter cycle may be increased, reduced, or unchanged under this circumstance. Of course sinus rhythm may be restored in some patients by digitalization alone or by combined therapy with quinidine and digitalis. By and large digitalization should be carried out first before quinidine is added when dealing with atrial flutter with 2:1 A-V response. Another important fact is that the serum digoxin level is often raised when digoxin and quinidine are given together.

The diagnosis of BFB consisting of RBBB and left anterior hemiblock can be made using the conventional criteria (*see* Case 7).

This ECG tracing was recorded postoperatively soon after aortic valve replacement for aortic stenosis on a 59-year-old man.

1. What is the cardiac rhythm diagnosis?

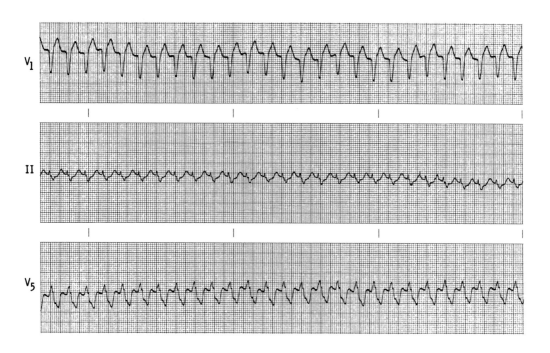

Diagnosis

The cardiac rhythm is supraventricular tachycardia, with a rate of 164 beats per minute. The cardiac cycle is precisely regular, with no discernible P waves.

Supraventricular tachycardia may be atrial, A-V junctional, or reciprocating tachycardia. In reality the P waves (either upright or inverted) may be superimposed to the T waves or the QRS complexes in supraventricular tachycardia so that the P waves may not be visible.

The diagnosis of LBBB can be established using the conventional criteria (see Case 33).

Clinically LBBB is a relatively common ECG abnormality in patients with aortic stenosis.

A 54-year-old man was admitted to the intermediate CCU because of CHF associated with rapid heart action. He was *not* taking any medication before this admission.

1. What is the cardiac rhythm diagnosis?
2. What is the proper therapeutic approach?

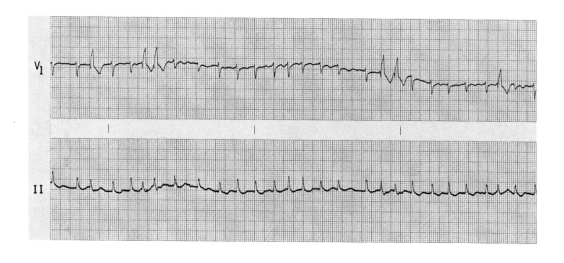

Diagnosis

The cardiac rhythm is AF, with very rapid ventricular response (ventricular rate: 160–200 beats per minute).

It is easy to recognize bizarre beats that sometimes occur consecutively. These bizarre beats represent aberrant ventricular conduction, which is initiated by Ashman's phenomenon in some areas (*see* Case 98).

The aberrantly conducted beats closely simulate VPCs, but a lack of postectopic pause excludes a possibility of VPCs (*see* Case 98).

Rapid digitalization is the treatment of choice for AF with rapid ventricular response.

This ECG tracing was obtained from a 72-year-old man with known COPD.

1. What is the cardiac rhythm diagnosis?
2. What is the ECG diagnosis?

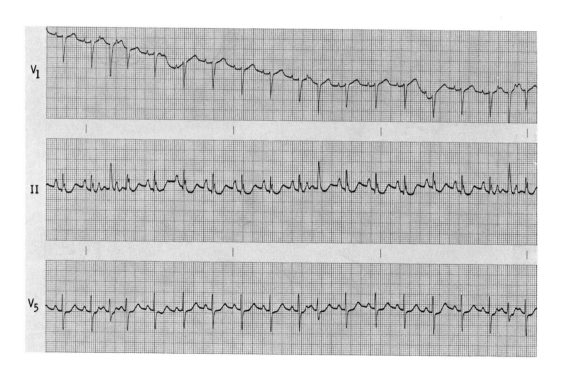

Diagnosis

The underlying cardiac rhythm is sinus ta-chycardia, with a rate of 102 beats per min-ute. There are frequent APCs, and some of them occur consecutively (atrial group beats).

It should be noted that some APCs are followed by bizarre QRS complexes (the 3rd and 18th beats). The reason for the ab-errant ventricular conduction is a very short coupling interval. The three common causes of aberrant ventricular conduction have been described previously (see Case 112).

It is easy to recognize tall and peaked P waves in lead II, indicative of RAH (P-pul-monale). The diagnostic criteria of RAH have been summarized previously (see Case 45). P-pulmonale is most commonly found in patients with COPD.

This ECG tracing was obtained from a 67-year-old man with palpitations. He was *not* taking any medication.

1. What is the cardiac rhythm diagnosis?
2. What is the proper therapeutic approach?

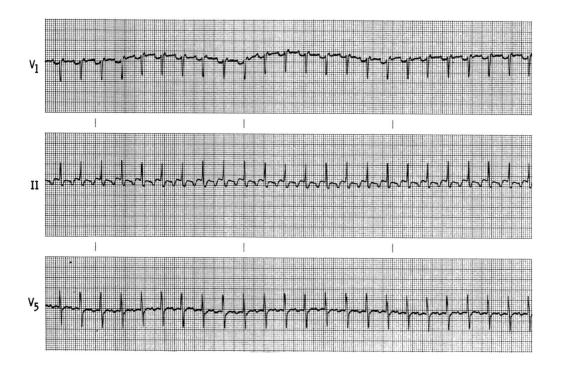

Diagnosis

The cardiac rhythm is atrial flutter (atrial rate: 290 beats per minute), with 2 : 1 A-V conduction (ventricular rate: 145 beats per minute).

Since all other flutter waves are superimposed to the terminal portions of the QRS complexes, the cardiac rhythm may easily be misinterpreted as A-V JT, AT, supraventricular tachycardia, or even sinus tachycardia.

Digitalization is the first choice of treatment for atrial flutter with 2 : 1 A-V conduction. When the clinical situation is urgent, DC shock should be applied immediately. Atrial flutter has been described in detail earlier (*see* Case 20).

A 51-year-old woman was brought to the ER because she suddenly developed a very rapid heart action associated with chest pain. She was *not* taking any drug.

1. What is the cardiac rhythm diagnosis?

2. What is the proper way of handling this arrhythmia?
3. What underlying disorder should be suspected first?

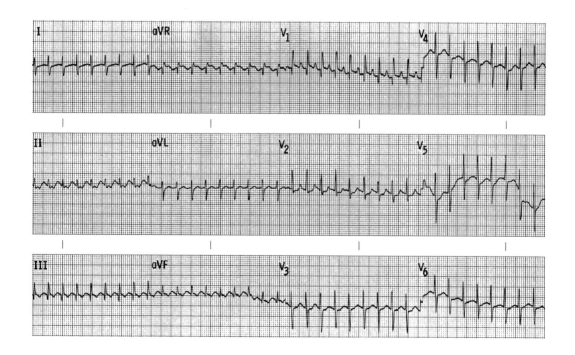

Diagnosis

The cardiac rhythm is supraventricular tachycardia, with a rate of 210 beats per minute. The cardiac cycle is precisely regular with no discernible P waves. Thus this supraventricular tachycardia may represent PAT, A-V JT, or reciprocating tachycardia.

As far as the ECG abnormality is concerned, there is incomplete RBBB pattern, with right axis deviation of the QRS complexes. In addition small Q waves in leads III and aVF suggest diaphragmatic MI.

When the above-mentioned ECG abnormalities with a very rapid supraventricular tachycardia associated with chest pain (especially pleuritic type) are interpreted together, pulmonary embolism should strongly be considered as an underlying disorder. S_1-Q_3 pattern is also present.

Various ECG abnormalities in pulmonary embolism are summarized as follows:

ECG Abnormalities in Pulmonary Embolism

1. Marked sinus tachycardia.
2. Various supraventricular tachyarrhythmias.
3. Right axis deviation of the QRS complexes.
4. RBBB (complete or incomplete).
5. P-pulmonale.
6. Pseudodiaphragmatic MI.
7. Inverted T waves in leads V_{1-3} (right ventricular strain pattern).
8. S_1-Q_3 pattern.
9. S_1-S_2-S_3 pattern.

One or more above-mentioned ECG findings may be observed in pulmonary embolism, but these ECG changes are often transient phenomena.

The first therapeutic approach is CSS. When CSS is found to be ineffective, various drugs may be tried (eg, digitalis, propranolol, verapamil), and often they are effective. If the clinical situation is extremely urgent, DC shock should be applied immediately. Then the patient should be treated in the intensive care unit for the conventional therapy for pulmonary embolism.

This ECG tracing was taken on a 68-year-old woman with COPD. She was *not* taking any cardiac drug.

1. What is the cardiac rhythm diagnosis?

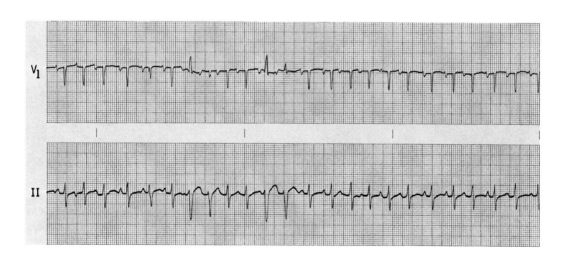

V_1

II

Diagnosis

The cardiac rhythm is MAT. It should be noted that there are many forms of P waves with varying PP cycles and varying PR intervals.

Some QRS complexes are bizarre because of aberrant ventricular conduction (*see* Case 98). The diagnostic criteria of MAT have been summarized previously (*see* Case 115).

As described earlier, MAT is most commonly encountered in patients with COPD. The aberrantly conducted beats closely simulate VPCs.

CASE 133

This ECG tracing, obtained from a 64-year-old woman, was presented to a weekly advanced arrhythmia conference.

1. What is the cardiac rhythm diagnosis?

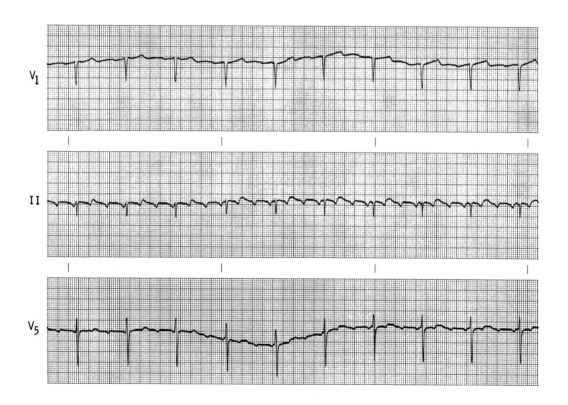

Diagnosis

At a glance the cardiac rhythm appears to be atrial flutter with 3 : 1 A-V block. Upon close observation, however, it becomes obvious that the FR intervals (the interval from the last flutter wave to the QRS complex) vary, but the RR intervals (ventricular cycles) remain constant, namely, the atrial activity is independent to the ventricular activity.

The correct rhythm diagnosis is atrial flutter (atrial rate: 190 beats per minute), with A-V JER (ventricular rate: 62 beats per minute) due to complete A-V block. Thus there is complete A-V dissociation.

The atrial flutter cycle is slower than usual because of quinidine effect.

There is left anterior hemiblock (see Case 27).

CASE 134

This is a routine ECG tracing taken on a 65-year-old man as a part of his annual checkup.

1. What is the cardiac rhythm diagnosis?

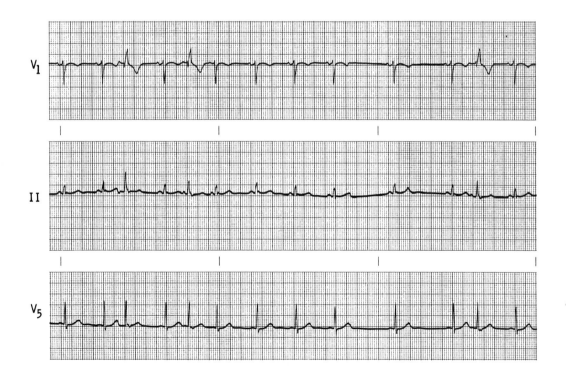

Diagnosis

The underlying cardiac rhythm is sinus (rate: 82 beats per minute), but there are frequent APCs.

It is interesting to note that some APCs show aberrant ventricular conduction, whereas some other APCs are blocked (nonconducted to the ventricles). In addition, some APCs occur consecutively, causing atrial group beats.

The blocked APCs superficially simulate sinus arrhythmia, S-A block, and sinus arrest. Aberrantly conducted APCs, of course, mimic VPCs. Aberrant ventricular conduction has been discussed in detail previously (*see* Case 98).

DI was suspected in a 72-year-old man with chronic CHF. This ECG tracing was discussed during a weekly arrhythmia conference.

1. What is the cardiac rhythm diagnosis?

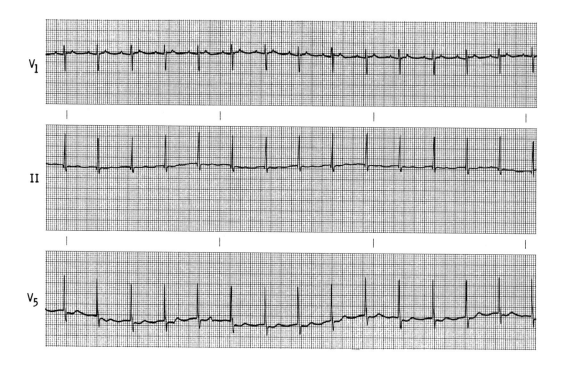

Diagnosis

The cardiac rhythm is AT (atrial rate: 184 beats per minute), with 2:1 A-V block (ventricular rate: 92 beats per minute). The PP cycles are regular, and all other P waves are conducted to the ventricles.

It has been shown that AT with A-V block is almost a pathognomonic feature of DI. Some cardiologists use the term "PAT with block" under this circumstance.

CASE 136

A 77-year-old woman with long-standing hypertension was admitted to the intermediate CCU because of acute CHF. She was *not* taking any medication regularly.

1. What is the cardiac rhythm diagnosis?
2. What is the proper therapeutic approach?

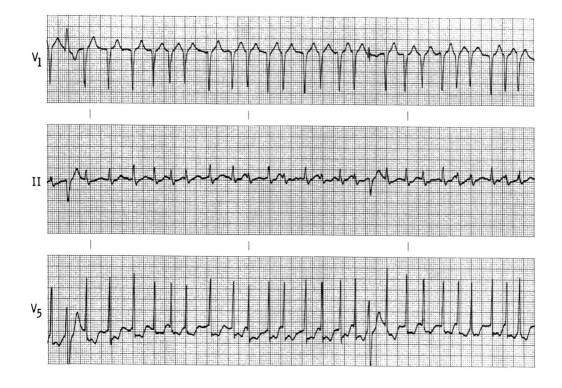

Diagnosis

The cardiac rhythm is AF, with very rapid ventricular response (ventricular rate: 150–200 beats per minute). Some QRS complexes are deformed in different degrees as a result of aberrant ventricular conduction (*see* Case 98). The aberrantly conducted beats closely simulate VPCs, but a lack of any postectopic pause excludes such a possibility.

Rapid digitalization is the treatment of choice for AF with rapid ventricular response whether or not there is CHF. Of course digitalis is more beneficial when AF is associated with CHF.

The diagnosis of LVH is established using the conventional diagnostic criteria (*see* Case 10).

CASE 137

This ECG tracing, obtained from a 64-year-old man, was discussed during a weekly arrhythmia conference.

1. What is the cardiac rhythm diagnosis?

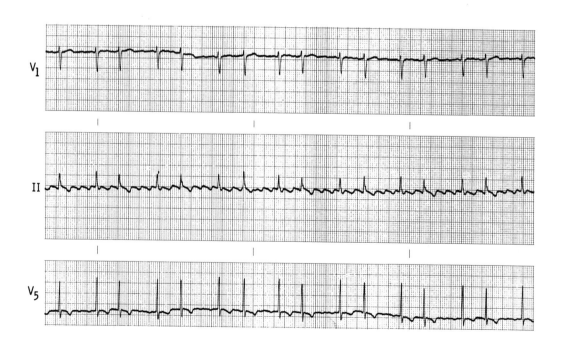

Diagnosis

The underlying cardiac rhythm is atrial flutter (atrial rate: 312 beats per minute). It is interesting to note a form of bigeminal rhythm, and each QRS complex is preceded by a flutter wave.

When this bigeminal rhythm is analyzed in-depth, the long RR interval is shorter than two short RR intervals. The long RR interval is shorter than four atrial flutter cycles, whereas the shorter RR interval is longer than two atrial flutter cycles. The FR interval is short after a longer RR interval, and the FR interval is longer during a shorter RR interval.

When these findings are interpreted together, atrial flutter with Wenckebach A-V conduction (the conduction ratio alternating between 2 : 1 and 4 : 1) can be established if any reader fully understands Wenckebach A-V block during sinus rhythm (see Case 82).

All other QRS complexes are slightly deformed because of aberrant ventricular conduction as a result of Ashman's phenomenon (see Case 98).

This ECG tracing was obtained from a 70-year-old woman who had been complaining of palpitations. She was *not* taking any medication.

1. What is the cardiac rhythm diagnosis?
2. What is the proper therapeutic approach?

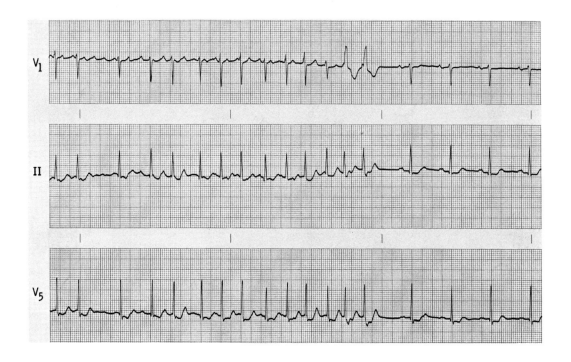

Diagnosis

The underlying cardiac rhythm is sinus (rate: 76 beats per minute), but atrial flutter-fibrillation occurs intermittently.

There are two bizarre QRS complexes just before a normal sinus rhythm is restored. It is *not* absolutely certain whether these bizarre beats represent aberrant ventricular conduction or VPCs because no ECG finding supports or excludes these possibilities. Nevertheless a possibility of aberrant ventricular conduction is greater judging from the configuration of the bizarre beats.

As far as the therapeutic approach is concerned, small amounts of digitalis (daily maintenance doses) may be effective in preventing recurrent atrial flutter-fibrillation. If digitalis alone is ineffective, oral quinidine may be added. In addition possible underlying causes (eg, excessive consumption of coffee or alcohol, emotional upset, hyperthyroidism) should be investigated and controlled.

This ECG tracing, taken on a 65-year-old man, was discussed during a weekly ECG conference.

1. What is the cardiac rhythm diagnosis?
2. What is the proper way of handling this patient?

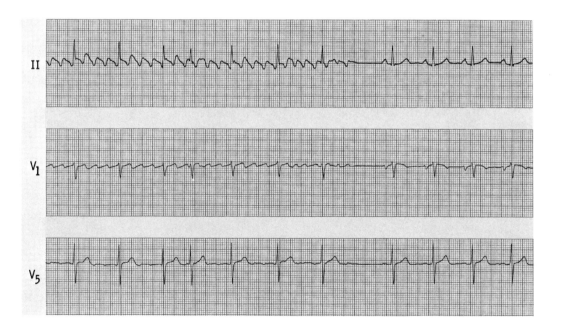

II

V₁

V₅

Diagnosis

The underlying cardiac rhythm is sinus (rate: 80 beats per minute), but atrial flutter (predominantly with 4 : 1 A-V block) occurs intermittently.

The therapeutic approach to intermittent atrial flutter is exactly the same as for intermittent AF or atrial flutter-fibrillation (*see* Case 138).

CASE 140

A 73-year-old woman was admitted to the intermediate CCU because she developed a rapid heart action during oral digitalis therapy. DI was considered. This ECG tracing was presented to the weekly advanced arrhythmia conference.

1. What is the cardiac rhythm diagnosis?
2. What is the proper way of handling this patient?

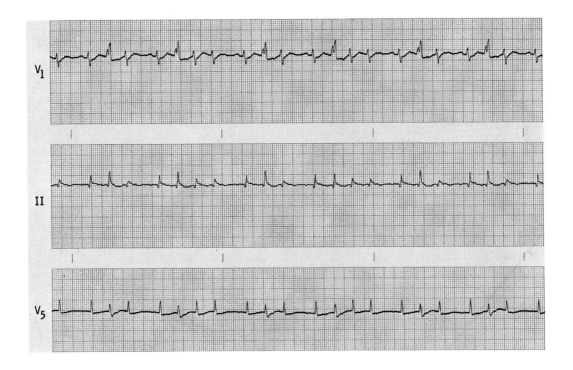

Diagnosis

Many inexperienced readers may erroneously diagnose this finding as AF with frequent VPCs because the cardiac rhythm is irregular and the P waves are not clearly visible. Bizarre beats appear to be VPCs to some inexperienced readers.

Upon close observation, however, rapidly occurring P waves may be recognized, and the ventricular cycle shows a regular irregularity, namely, the correct rhythm diagnosis is AT (atrial rate: 180 beats per minute), with Wenckebach A-V block (the conduction ratios vary from 4 : 3 to 5 : 4) and frequent aberrant ventricular conduction. The aberrant ventricular conduction occurs as a result of Ashman's phenomenon (see Case 98). The P waves are best seen in lead V_1.

The proper therapeutic approach to DI has been described earlier (see Case 82).

Old diaphragmatic and posterior MI is considered.

CASE 141

A 70-year-old woman was brought to the ER because she developed a rapid heart action suddenly. She was *not* taking any medication.

  1. What is the cardiac rhythm diagnosis?

2. What is the ECG diagnosis?
3. What is the proper therapeutic approach?

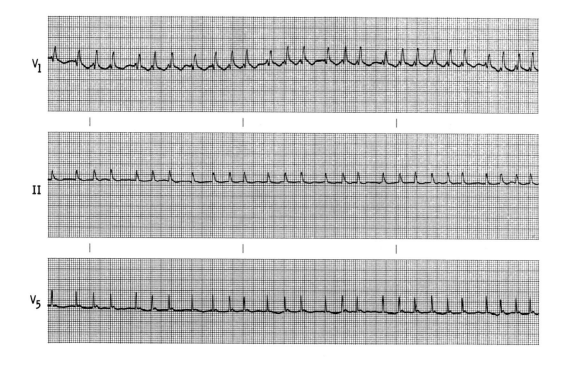

Diagnosis

The cardiac rhythm is AF, with a very rapid ventricular response (ventricular rate: 170–195 beats per minute).

The diagnosis of incomplete RBBB can be made without any difficulty using the conventional criteria (*see* Case 34).

The best therapeutic approach to AF with rapid ventricular response is rapid digitalization.

This ECG tracing, obtained from a 61-year-old man, was discussed during a weekly student ECG conference.

1. What is the cardiac rhythm diagnosis?

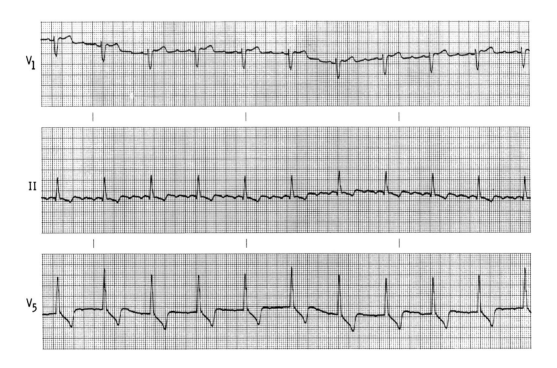

Diagnosis

The cardiac rhythm is atrial flutter (atrial rate: 260 beats per minute), with 4 : 1 A-V block (ventricular rate: 65 beats per minute). The ventricular cycle is precisely regular because every fourth atrial flutter waves are conducted to the ventricles.

The diagnosis of LVH is considered, although the voltage is insufficient for the criteria (*see* Case 10).

CASE 143

This ECG tracing was obtained from a 28-year-old woman with RHD. She was *not* taking any cardiac drug.

1. What is the cardiac rhythm diagnosis?
2. What is the proper therapeutic approach?

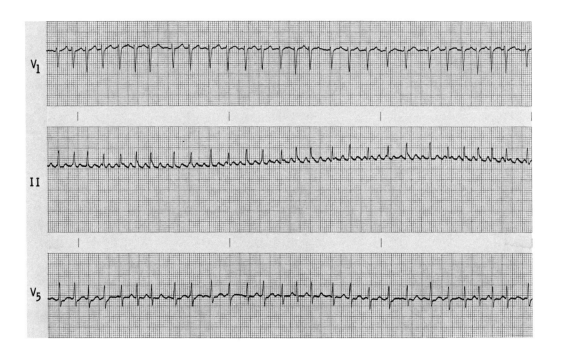

Diagnosis

At a glance the cardiac rhythm appears to be AF with a rapid ventricular response. However, regularly occurring atrial flutter cycles can be identified upon close observation. It should be noted, however, that the flutter cycle is faster (atrial rate: 450 beats per minute) than the usual atrial flutter (usual atrial rate: 250–350 beats per minute). The term "atrial impure flutter" is applied when dealing with rapid atrial flutter cycles (atrial rate: 350–450 beats per minute).

Clinically atrial impure flutter is very similar to AF or atrial flutter. Thus the therapeutic approach is also the same (*see* Cases 9 and 20). Rapid digitalization is the treatment of choice.

Digitalis toxicity was suspected in a 72-year-old man who developed a new cardiac arrhythmia during oral digitalis therapy associated with worsening of his CHF.

1. What is the cardiac rhythm diagnosis?

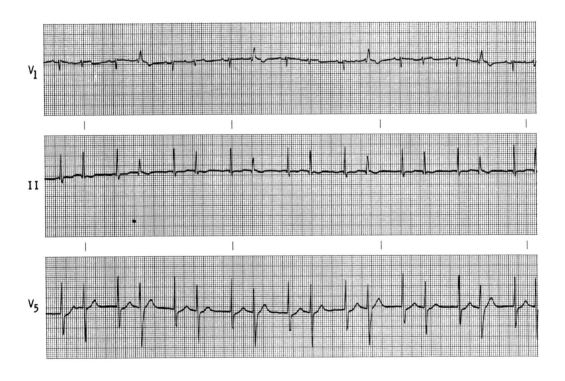

Diagnosis

The cardiac rhythm is AT (atrial rate: 162 beats per minute), with 3:2 Wenckebach A-V block and frequent aberrant ventricular conduction. The aberrant ventricular conduction of varying degree occurs as a result of Ashman's phenomenon (*see* Case 98).

The P waves are best shown in lead V$_1$, and the ventricular cycle exhibits a regular irregularity. For better understanding of this arrhythmia all readers should study Wenckebach A-V block during sinus rhythm (*see* Case 82).

It has been well documented that AT with A-V block (usually Wenckebach type) is one of the commonest arrhythmias induced by digitalis (*see* Case 82).

CASE 145

This ECG tracing, obtained from a 74-year-old man, was discussed during a weekly arrhythmia conference.

1. What is the cardiac rhythm diagnosis?

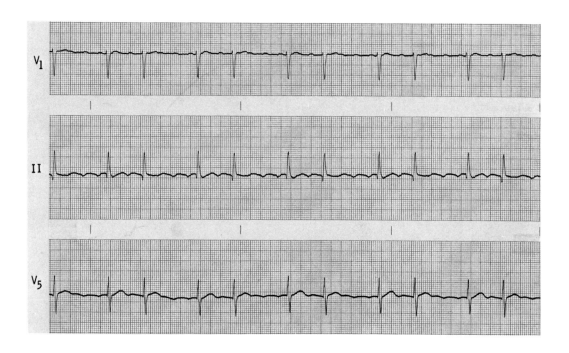

Diagnosis

The cardiac rhythm exhibits a form of bigeminal rhythm, and the underlying atrial mechanism is atrial flutter, namely, the rhythm diagnosis is atrial flutter (atrial rate: 200 beats per minute) with Wenckebach A-V block. The A-V conduction ratios alternate between 2 : 1 and 4 : 1. Detailed explanation of an atrial flutter with Wenckebach A-V conduction is found elsewhere (*see* Case 137). If any reader has difficulty in understanding Wenckebach A-V block in atrial flutter, he or she should study Wenckebach A-V block during sinus rhythm (*see* Case 82) in-depth.

As described repeatedly, atrial flutter cycle is often reduced by quinidine or quinidine-like drugs.

This ECG tracing, which belongs to an 83-year-old man with chronic AF, was discussed during a weekly advanced arrhythmia conference. By reviewing his previous ECG tracings, the QRS complexes have been always normal.

1. What is the cardiac rhythm diagnosis?

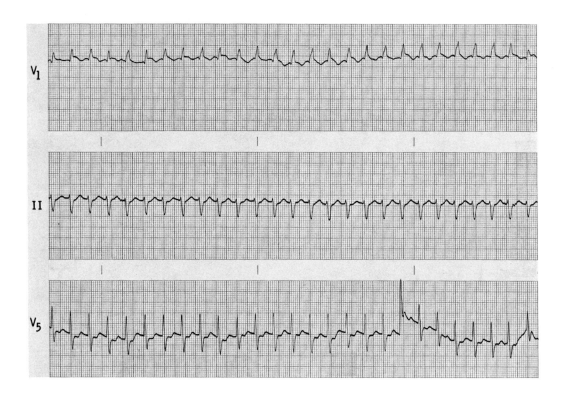

Diagnosis

The ventricular cycle is precisely regular, and there are no discernible P waves. The QRS configuration demonstrates a BFB pattern consisting of incomplete RBBB and left anterior hemiblock. Remember that this patient always had normal QRS complexes during AF.

When the above-mentioned findings are carefully analyzed, some experienced readers may be able to make the diagnosis of AF with fascicular tachycardia (rate: 175 beats per minute), producing complete A-V dissociation. Judging from the configuration of the QRS complexes (incomplete RBBB with left anterior hemiblock pattern), the tachycardia is most likely arising from the left posterior fascicle of the left bundle branch system.

In general, the fascicular tachycardia is a form of VT.

CHAPTER SEVEN

ATRIOVENTRICULAR JUNCTIONAL ARRHYTHMIAS

CASE 147

An 83-year-old man suddenly developed a rapid heart action. He was *not* taking any drug.

1. What is the cardiac rhythm diagnosis?
2. What is the proper way of handling this arrhythmia?

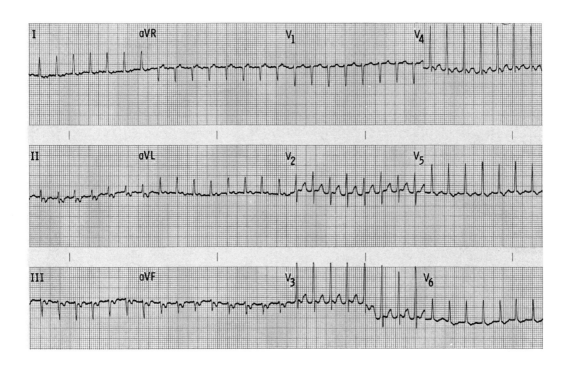

Diagnosis

The cardiac rhythm diagnosis is paroxysmal A-V JT, with a rate of 175 beats per minute. The cardiac cycle is precisely regular, and each QRS complex is followed by a retrograde P wave. An alternative diagnosis is reciprocating (re-entrant) tachycardia.

In A-V JT or rhythm, a retrograde P wave may precede or follow each QRS complex depending upon the sequence of the atrial and ventricular activation. When the atria are activated simultaneously with the ventricular activation, a retrograde P wave will be superimposed to the QRS complex leading to absent P wave. When there is A-V dissociation, of course, the P waves and the QRS complexes will be independent. Needless to say, there will be no P waves when the atrial mechanism is AF or atrial flutter.

The clinical significance of paroxysmal A-V JT is very similar to that of PAT. The therapeutic approach is also very similar under these circumstances. CSS is often effective in terminating paroxysmal A-V JT. Otherwise various drugs (eg, digoxin, beta blockers) may be tried, and they are also very effective. DC shock is applied only when the clinical circumstance is extremely urgent (eg, very rapid rate). EPS is considered when the tachycardia becomes refractory to the conventional therapy.

As far as the underlying causes of paroxysmal A-V JT are concerned, any unusual personal habits (eg, excessive consumption of coffee or alcohol, emotional stress) should be investigated and controlled if possible. Other possible underlying disorders may include hyperthyroidism, MVPs, and WPW syndrome (see Chapter 9).

CASE 148

This ECG tracing was obtained from a 76-year-old man during oral digitalis therapy. DI was considered.

1. What is the cardiac rhythm diagnosis?
2. What is the ECG diagnosis?

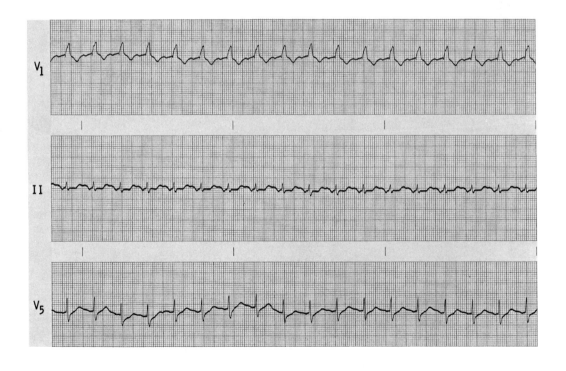

Diagnosis

The cardiac rhythm is nonparoxysmal A-V JT, with a rate of 115 beats per minute.

The cardiac cycle is precisely regular, and each QRS complex is preceded by a retrograde P wave.

The diagnosis of RBBB is obvious using the conventional criteria (*see* Case 34).

Although almost every known cardiac arrhythmia may be induced by DI, nonparoxysmal A-V JT is probably one of the commonest rhythm disturbances in DI.

CASE 149

A 74-year-old woman was admitted to the CCU because acute MI was diagnosed.

1. What is the cardiac rhythm diagnosis?

2. What is the ECG diagnosis?

3. What is the proper way of handling this arrhythmia?

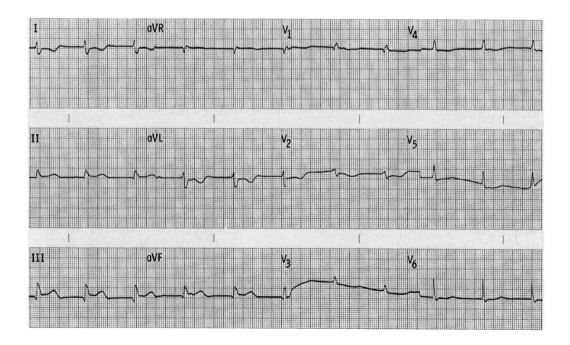

Diagnosis

The cardiac rhythm is A-V JER, with a rate of 58 beats per minute. The cardiac cycle is precisely regular, but there are no discernible P waves.

The diagnosis of acute diaphragmatic (inferior) MI is made on the basis of pathologic Q waves in leads II, III, and aVF, with ST segment elevation. In addition there is RBBB (see Case 34).

In most cases with acute diaphragmatic MI, sinus rhythm is restored within two to three days without any active treatment. When A-V JER persists more than 1 week under this circumstance, however, dysfunctioning sinus node (SSS) should be considered. Artificial pacing is strongly considered when the A-V JER persists and the patient becomes symptomatic (eg, syncope or near syncope, see Case 89).

CASE 150

An 81-year-old man was brought to the ER because he experienced frequent episodes of syncope and near syncope. He was *not* taking any medication.

1. What is the cardiac rhythm diagnosis?

2. What is most likely the underlying disorder?
3. What is the proper way of handling this patient?

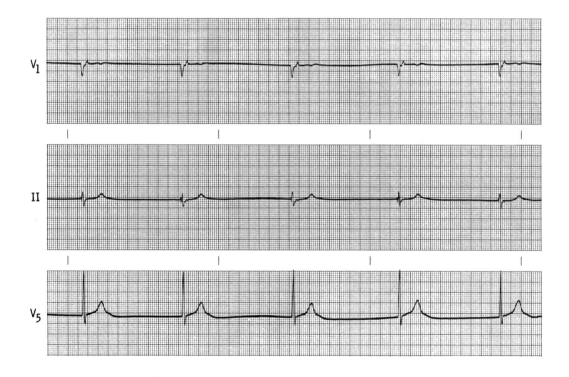

Diagnosis

The ventricular rate is extremely slow (28 beats per minute), and the cardiac cycle is precisely regular. Each QRS complex is followed by a retrograde P wave, and the QRS complex is normal (narrow). When these ECG findings are interpreted together, the cardiac rhythm is a very slow A-V JER with a rate of 28 beats per minute. It is possible, however, that the escape rhythm may be arising from the His bundle in considering a very slow heart rate. On the other hand, A-V JER may be much slower than usual in patients with SSS because the diseased sinus node often coexists with diseased A-V node.

The underlying disorder is most likely advanced SSS for which permanent artificial pacing is definitely indicated (see Case 89).

CASE 151

This ECG tracing was taken on a 52-year-old woman with chronic CHF. DI was suspected.

1. What is the cardiac rhythm diagnosis?

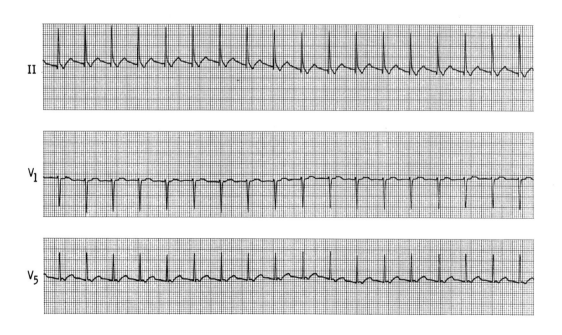

II

V₁

V₅

Diagnosis

The cardiac rhythm is nonparoxysmal A-V JT, with a rate of 116 beats per minute. The cardiac cycle is precisely regular, and each QRS complex is followed by a retrograde P wave. The QRS complexes are normal (narrow).

In A-V JT the retrograde P wave may precede or follow each QRS complex depending upon the sequence of atrial and ventricular activation (*see* Case 147). Obviously the atrial activation follows the ventricular activation in this ECG tracing.

The usual heart rates in nonparox-ysmal A-V JT range from 70–130 beats per minute—the same rate ranges as sinus rhythm.

Nonparoxysmal A-V JT most commonly occurs in patients with acute diaphragmatic MI and DI. Less commonly this arrhythmia may be observed during the immediate postoperative period following various open heart surgeries and in patients with myocarditis or cardiomyopathy. By and large nonparoxysmal A-V JT is very unusual in healthy people.

CASE 152

This ECG tracing, obtained from a 72-year-old man, was discussed during a weekly ECG conference.

1. What is the cardiac rhythm diagnosis?
2. What is the ECG diagnosis?

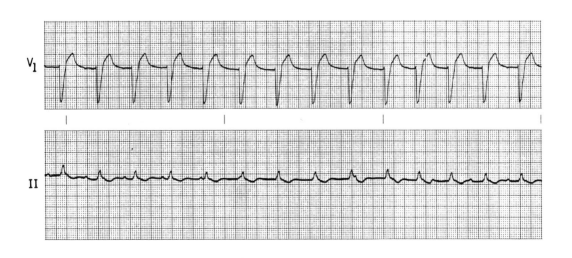

Diagnosis

The underlying cardiac rhythm is sinus (atrial rate: 84 beats per minute) with first degree A-V block, but nonparoxysmal A-V JT occurs intermittently (ventricular rate: 90 beats per minute), leading to incomplete A-V dissociation.

Slow VT (nonparoxysmal VT or accelerated idioventricular rhythm) is closely simulated because the QRS complexes are broad, and the ventricular cycle is regular in most areas (see Chapter 8). Upon close observation regularly occurring sinus P waves are recognizable, and A-V dissociation is present in most areas.

Needless to say, the QRS complexes are broad because of LBBB (see Case 33).

CASE 153

This ECG tracing was taken on a 60-year-old woman with chronic CHF.

1. What is the cardiac rhythm diagnosis?
2. What is the ECG diagnosis?

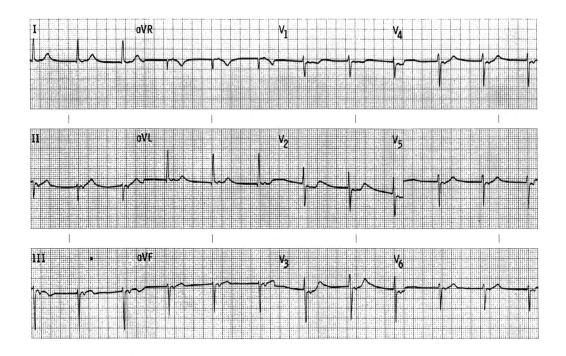

Diagnosis

The cardiac rhythm is nonparoxysmal A-V JT, with a rate of 64 beats per minute. It should be noted that each QRS complex is followed by a retrograde P wave. The finding indicates that the ventricular activation precedes the atrial activation (see Case 147).

The diagnosis of left anterior hemiblock is made using the conventional criteria (see Case 27).

SSS should strongly be considered when A-V JER or a relatively slow nonparoxysmal A-V JT persists for a long period of time as a chronic form (see Case 89).

CASE 154

This ECG tracing was obtained from a 68-year-old man soon after CABS.

1. What is the cardiac rhythm diagnosis?
2. What is the proper way of handling this arrhythmia?

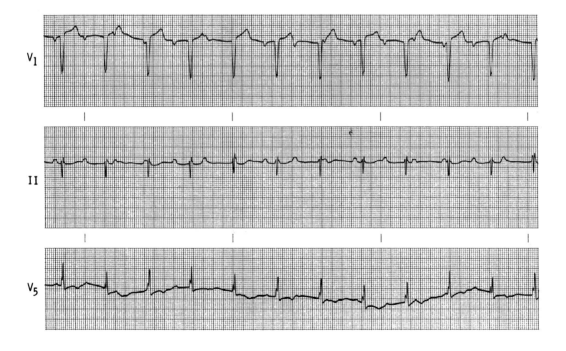

Diagnosis

The underlying atrial mechanism is sinus (atrial rate: 100 beats per minute), but non-paroxysmal A-V JT is present (ventricular rate: 68 beats per minute), independent of the atrial activity, leading to complete A-V dissociation.

The diagnosis of incomplete LBBB as well as LAH is considered (*see* Cases 27 and 33).

Nonparoxysmal A-V JT is *not* uncommon soon after various open cardiac surgeries, but this arrhythmia is usually self-limited and transient. Thus no treatment is necessary in most cases.

CASE 155

This ECG tracing, taken on a 70-year-old woman, was discussed during a weekly advanced arrhythmia conference.

   1. What is the cardiac rhythm diagnosis?

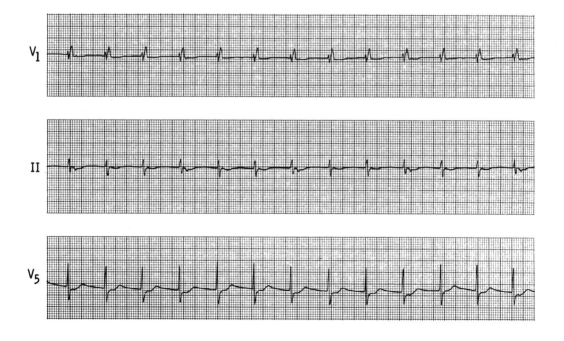

Diagnosis

The cardiac rhythm diagnosis is nonparoxysmal A-V JT, with a rate of 92 beats per minute. It is extremely interesting to note that a retrograde atrial activation occurs only on every third beat. Thus a complete rhythm diagnosis is nonparoxysmal A-V JT with 3 : 1 V-A block.

The diagnosis of incomplete RBBB is made using the conventional criteria (*see* Case 34).

Remember that in a pure form of A-V JT a retrograde P wave may precede or follow *each* QRS complex (*see* Cases 147 and 148). At times no P wave is discernible when the atrial and ventricular activation occurs simultaneously (*see* Case 147).

DI was suspected in a 76-year-old woman.

1. What is the cardiac rhythm diagnosis?
2. What is the ECG diagnosis?

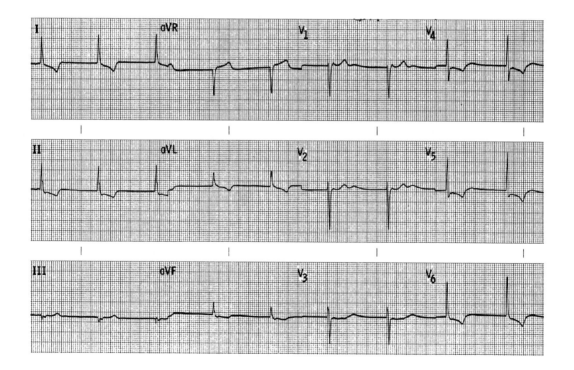

Diagnosis

The cardiac rhythm is A-V JER with a rate of 52 beats per minute. It should be noted that each QRS complex is followed by a retrograde P wave. Many inexperienced readers may not recognize the retrograde P waves because they are superimposed to the end portion of the QRS complexes.

The diagnosis of LVH is obvious using the conventional criteria (*see* Case 10).

Another important ECG abnormality in this tracing is prominent U waves, most pronounced in leads V_{2-4}. It has been stressed that hypokalemia commonly predisposes to DI, and the earliest sign of hypokalemia is prominent U waves (*see* Case 82).

Incomplete RBBB is superficially simulated because the retrograde P waves are superimposed to the end portion of the QRS complexes so that the QRS complex appear to be RR' in leads V_{1-2}.

CASE 157

This ECG tracing was obtained from a 73-year-old woman with a permanent artificial pacemaker. This tracing was discussed during a weekly complex arrhythmia conference. DI was considered.

1. What is the cardiac rhythm diagnosis?

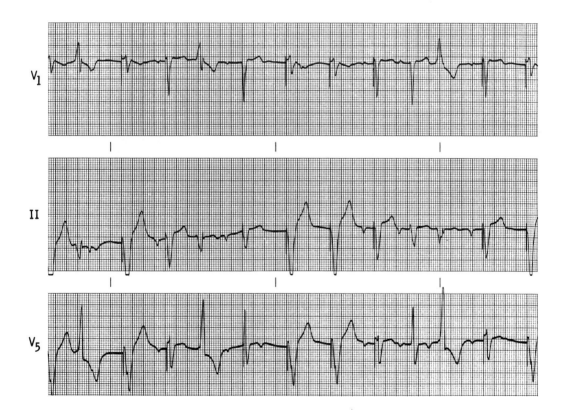

Diagnosis

The underlying atrial mechanism is non-paroxysmal A-V JT, with a rate of 92 beats per minute. It is interesting to note that some expected retrograde P waves are absent because of intermittent exit block.

The ventricular activity is controlled primarily by a demand ventricular pacemaker, but there are frequent VPCs (the 2nd, 5th, and 11th beats).

In addition there are frequent ventricular fusion beats (the 4th, 6th, 9th, and 12th beats).

There is only one conducted A-V junc-tional beat (the tenth beat). All of the above-mentioned ventricular fusion beats represent the mixed beats between the A-V JT beats and the ventricular pacemaker beats.

In summary, the complete rhythm diagnosis is nonparoxysmal A-V JT with intermittent exit block and intermittent demand ventricular pacemaker rhythm with frequent ventricular fusion beats producing incomplete A-V dissociation associated with frequent VPCs.

CHAPTER EIGHT

VENTRICULAR ARRHYTHMIAS

This ECG tracing was taken on a 70-year-old hypertensive male who had been suffering from chronic CHF for many years.

1. What is the cardiac rhythm diagnosis?

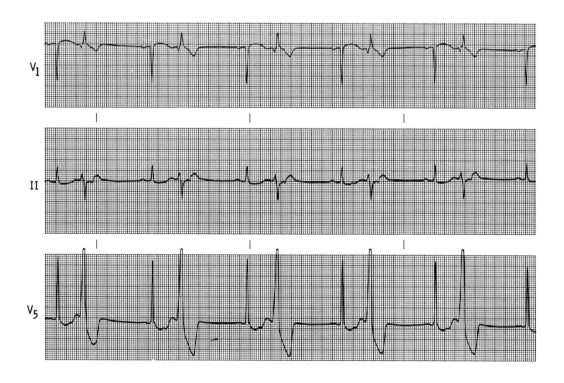

Diagnosis

The underlying cardiac rhythm is sinus, but there are frequent VPCs, producing ventricular bigeminy. It is interesting to note that each VPC is followed by a retrograde P wave, meaning atrial capture.

By and large a VPC is followed by a full compensatory pause because the sinus PP cycle is *not* disturbed by the ectopic ventricular impulse. In other words, the sinus node automaticity is *not* disturbed by a VPC in most cases. On rare occasions, however, a VPC may be followed by a retrograde P wave when the ventricular ectopic impulse activates the atria in a retrograde fashion following the ventricular activation. In other rare cases a VPC may be interpolated, meaning that the VPC is sandwiched between two consecutively occurring sinus beats (*see* Case 159).

Various ECG findings that support ventricular ectopy are summarized as follows:

ECG Findings That Support (or Favor) Ventricular Ectopy

- Full compensatory pause during sinus rhythm (occasionally interpolated)—no disturbance on the sinus PP cycle.
- Significant pause after a bizarre QRS complex in AF or flutter.
- No premature P wave preceding a bizarre QRS complex.
- Extremely broad and bizarre QRS complex.
- No evidence of Ashman's phenomenon.
- LBBB pattern or multiformed.
- Bizarre QRS complex in elderly or cardiac patients and/or in digitalis toxicity.

The above-mentioned ECG findings that support or favor the ventricular ectopy are very important to understand because aberrant ventricular conduction often closely simulates ventricular ectopy (*see* Case 98).

The diagnosis of LVH is obvious using the conventional diagnostic criteria (*see* Case 10).

CASE 159

This ECG tracing, obtained from a 60-year-old man, was discussed during a weekly student ECG conference.

1. What is the cardiac rhythm diagnosis?

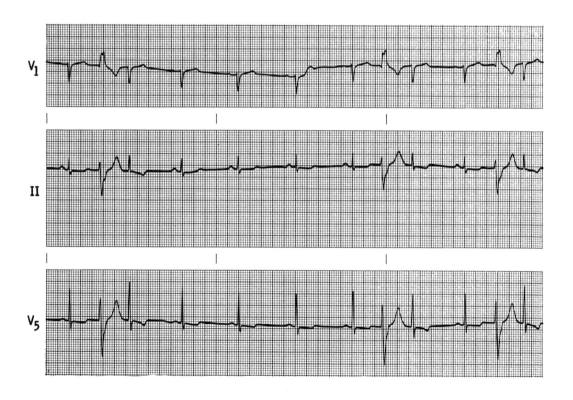

Diagnosis

The underlying cardiac rhythm is sinus (rate: 60 beats per minute), but there are frequent VPCs that are interpolated, namely, a VPC occurs between two consecutively occurring sinus beats without any pause. Remember that a VPC is almost always followed by a full compensatory pause (*see* Case 158).

Another interesting ECG finding is a deformed T wave of the sinus beat immedi- ately following a VPC. This finding is termed "postectopic T wave change." The postectopic T wave change seems to occur more commonly in patients with significant organic heart disease. In addition the postectopic T wave change is much commoner following an interpolated VPC than an ordinary VPC with a full compensatory pause.

CASE 160

A 33-year-old woman with multiple risk factors for CAD was admitted to the CCU because of acute MI.

1. What is the cardiac rhythm diagnosis?
2. What is the proper therapeutic approach?

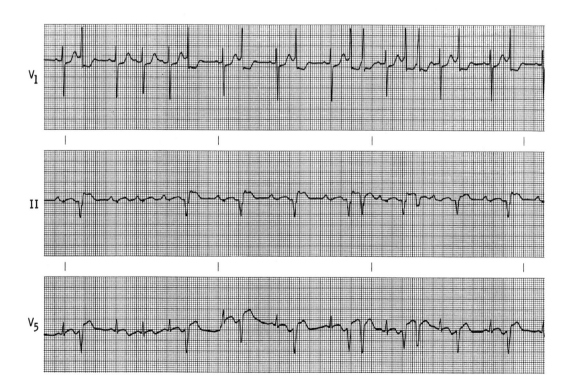

Diagnosis

The underlying cardiac rhythm is sinus tachycardia, with a rate of 115 beats per minute. There are frequent VPCs, and some of them occur consecutively leading to ventricular group beats. Some VPCs are interpolated.

The term "R-on-T phenomenon" is used when any cardiac impulse (often VPC) is superimposed to the top of the T wave of the preceding beat. The R-on-T phenomenon is important to recognize because the incidence of VF is greater because the threshold of the VF is low during the vulnerable period of the ventricles corresponding to the duration of the T wave.

The R-on-T phenomenon is often observed in patients with acute MI, especially when the coupling interval is very short or the QT interval is prolonged.

By and large *VPCs are considered to be clinically serious* in the following circumstances:

Clinically Serious VPCs

1. VPCs in acute MI or any other active heart disease.
2. Frequent VPCs (30 or more per hour).
3. Multifocal VPCs.
4. Grouped VPCs.
5. VPCs with R-on-T phenomenon.
6. VPCs following termination of VT or VF.
7. VPCs easily provoked by exercise or electrical stimulation (EPS).

This patient's VPCs are considered to be serious because of the presence of acute MI and frequent multifocal and grouped VPCs with the R-on-T phenomenon.

In addition to the usual acute coronary care, intravenous lidocaine should be the first drug of choice for the patient's VPCs. If lidocaine is found to be ineffective, all other antiarrhythmic agents (eg, amiodarone, procainamide) should be tried.

CASE 161

This ECG tracing was obtained from a 76-year-old man with DI.

1. What is the cardiac rhythm diagnosis?

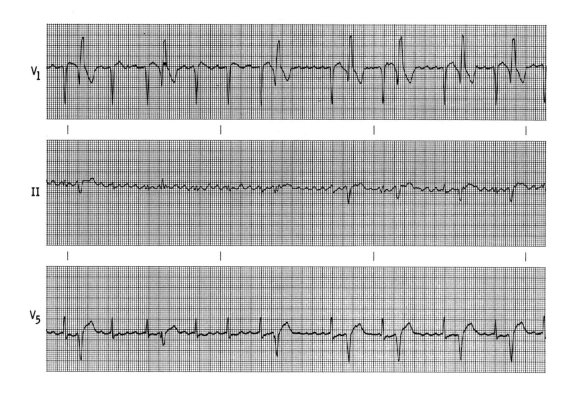

Diagnosis

The underlying cardiac rhythm is atrial flutter-fibrillation, but there are frequent VPCs.

The R-on-T phenomenon is observed because the coupling interval of the VPC is very short. As described previously (*see* Case 160), VPCs with the R-on-T phenomenon predispose to VF.

In addition to discontinuation of digitalis, VPCs induced by digitalis are best treated with phenytoin (Dilantin). When the serum potassium is found to be very low, however, administration of potassium may be even more effective under this circumstance.

These cardiac rhythm strips were recorded from a 71-year-old man with CAD (previous history of diaphragmatic MI). He was *not* taking any medication.

1. What is the cardiac rhythm diagnosis?
2. What is the proper way of handling this patient?

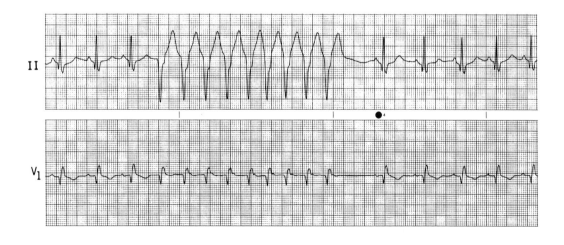

Diagnosis

The underlying cardiac rhythm is sinus, but VT occurs intermittently with a rate of 166 beats per minute.

There is a significant pause following termination of VT.

Since the configuration of the sinus beats closely resembles the VT beats in lead V_1, some inexperienced readers may misdiagnose the finding as supraventricular tachycardia.

The diagnosis of RBBB is obvious using the conventional criteria (*see* Case 34).

Intravenous lidocaine is the first drug of choice for paroxysmal VT. When lidocaine is found to be ineffective, other antiarrhythmic agents (eg, amiodarone, procainamide) should be tried. If VT persists as a sustained VT, DC shock should be tried. EPS is considered only when VT becomes refractory to the conventional drug therapy.

This ECG tracing, taken on a 76-year-old man, was discussed during a weekly arrhythmia conference.

1. What is the cardiac rhythm diagnosis?
2. What is the ECG diagnosis?

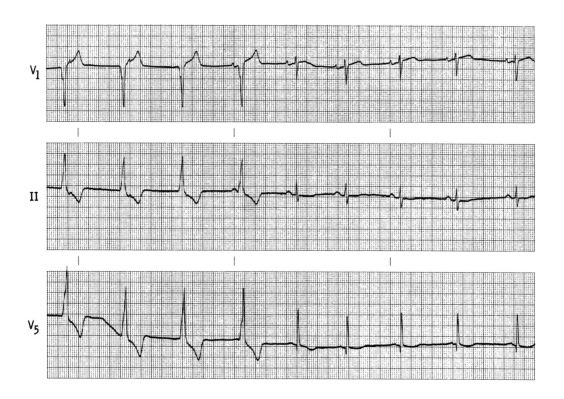

Diagnosis

The underlying cardiac rhythm is sinus bradycardia with arrhythmia (rate: 53–60 beats per minute), but there are four bizarre beats in the first half of the tracing, namely, there is intermittent VER with a rate of 53 beats per minute, leading to incomplete A-V dissociation. The ventricular rate is somewhat faster than usual because the VER is slightly accelerated. The usual rates of the VER range from 25–40 beats per minute.

The fourth beat represents a ventricular fusion beat (a mixed beat between the sinus and the ventricular escape beats).

LAH and old lateral MI are considered (*see* Case 33).

CASE 164

This ECG tracing was obtained from a 78-year-old man with known CAD.

1. What is the cardiac rhythm diagnosis?
2. What is the ECG diagnosis?

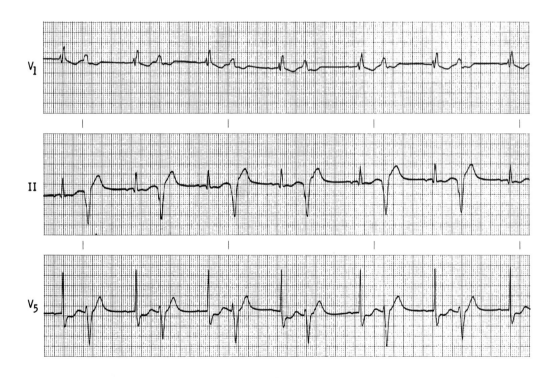

Diagnosis

The underlying cardiac rhythm is non-paroxysmal A-V JT, with a rate of 80 beats per minute. Note that there are frequent VPCs producing ventricular bigeminy. The P waves are inverted in lead II, meaning a retrograde conduction of the atrial activation.

The diagnosis of RBBB is obvious using the conventional criteria (*see* Case 34). In addition old diaphragmatic-posterior MI is considered.

CASE 165

This ECG tracing, which was taken on an 84-year-old man, was discussed during a weekly arrhythmia conference.

    1. What is the cardiac rhythm diagnosis?

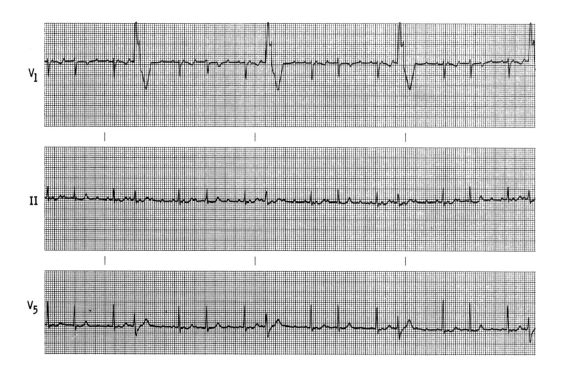

Diagnosis

The underlying cardiac rhythm is atrial flutter (atrial rate: 300 beats per minute), but the ventricular cycle exhibits a regular irregularity, namely, the rhythm diagnosis is atrial flutter, with Wenckebach A-V conduction (A-V conduction ratios alternate between 4 : 1 and 2 : 1). Detailed explanation regarding Wenckebach A-V conduction in atrial flutter is found in Case 137. For better understanding of atrial flutter with Wenckebach A-V conduction, all readers should study Wenckebach A-V block during sinus rhythm (see Case 82).

In addition there are frequent VPCs producing ventricular quadrigeminy.

CASE 166

A 65-year-old woman with known CAD developed a rapid heart action. She had suffered from at least two MIs in the past.

1. What is the cardiac rhythm diagnosis?
2. What is the proper way of handling this patient?

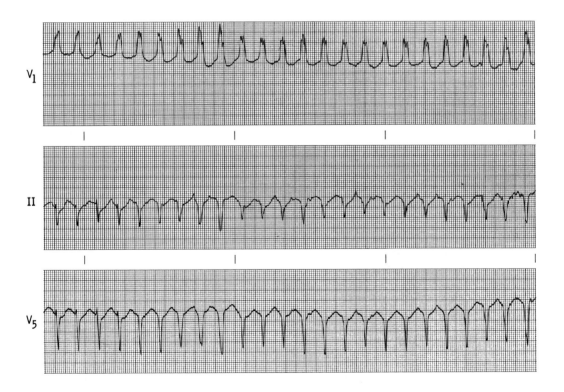

V₁

II

V₅

Diagnosis

At a glance the atrial activity is not discernible. However, regularly occurring P waves can be appreciated upon close observation, with a rate of 187 beats per minute, namely, AT is present in the atria (rate: 187 beats per minute). The P waves are best seen in lead II. Independently, VT is present in the ventricles, with a rate of 150 beats per minute. Thus complete A-V dissociation is produced.

When the above-mentioned ECG findings are interpreted together, this tracing demonstrates AT (atrial rate: 187 beats per minute) with VT (ventricular rate: 150 beats per minute), producing complete A-V dissociation.

The drug of choice for VT is intravenous injection of lidocaine. If lidocaine is ineffective, other antiarrhythmic agents such as procainamide and amiodarone should be tried. When the clinical situation is urgent, DC shock should be applied immediately. EPS should strongly be considered when the conventional therapy fails to terminate VT or when VT recurs.

A 67-year-old man was admitted to the CCU because of acute diaphragmatic (inferior) MI. This ECG tracing was discussed during a weekly advanced arrhythmia conference.

1. What is the cardiac rhythm diagnosis?
2. What is the proper therapeutic approach?

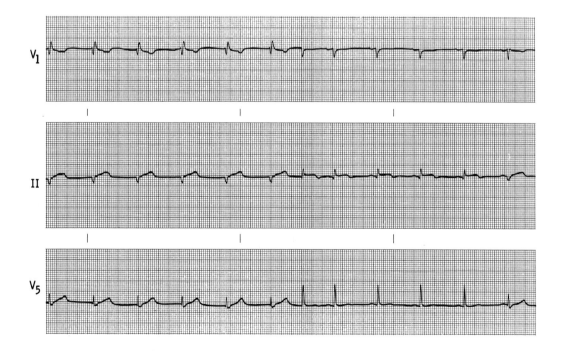

Diagnosis

The underlying cardiac rhythm is sinus, with a rate of 72 beats per minute. A first half of the tracing reveals an ectopic rhythm with a rate of 70 beats per minute, producing incomplete A-V dissociation. The QRS complex shows incomplete RBBB pattern with left anterior hemiblock pattern. Thus the ectopic rhythm represents left posterior fascicular tachycardia. In a broad sense the fascicular tachycardia is a form of idioventricular tachycardia (accelerated idioventricular rhythm or nonparoxysmal VT).

As far as the therapeutic approach is concerned, the fascicular tachycardia is a self-limited and transient arrhythmia. Thus no active treatment is necessary in most cases.

The diagnosis of acute diaphragmatic MI is obvious (abnormal Q waves with ST segment elevation and T wave inversion in leads II, III, and aVF (only lead II is shown here).

CHAPTER NINE

WOLFF-PARKINSON-WHITE SYNDROME

This ECG tracing was taken on a 23-year-old man with occasional episodes of palpitations. He was *not* taking any medication and was found to be healthy otherwise.

1. What is the ECG diagnosis?
2. What is the proper way of handling this patient?

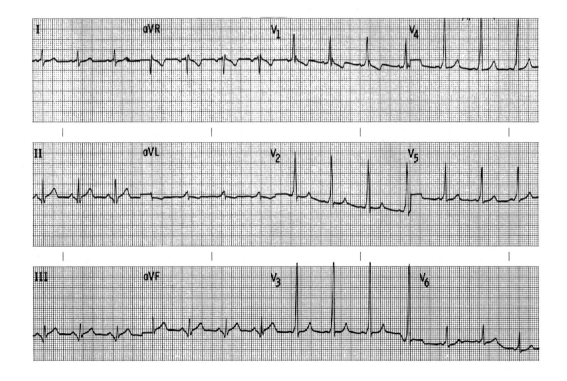

Diagnosis

The cardiac rhythm is sinus, with a rate of 80 beats per minute.

The diagnosis of WPW syndrome can be made by most experienced readers using the conventional criteria:

Diagnostic Criteria of WPW Syndrome

- Initial slurring of the QRS complexes (delta waves).
- Short PR interval due to a delta wave.
- Broad QRS complex due to a delta wave.
- Secondary T wave change (*not* always present).

It has been well documented that any individual with WPW syndrome is prone to develop various tachyarrhythmias. The commonest tachyarrhythmia in WPW syndrome is a reciprocating tachycardia (*see* Case 172). Less commonly, AF or atrial flutter may occur in this syndrome (*see* Case 175). During the above-mentioned tachyarrhythmias, the QRS complexes may be normal when the cardiac impulses are conducted to the ventricles via the normal A-V conduction system (*see* Case 172). On the other hand, the QRS complexes are broad and bizarre when the cardiac impulses are conducted to the ventricles via an anomalous pathway (*see* Case 175).

When the patient experiences episodic palpitations, the Holter monitor ECG should be taken to document the tachyarrhythmia. For reciprocating tachycardia with normal QRS complexes (*see* Case 172), various drugs such as beta blockers, calcium blockers (eg, verapamil), and digoxin are very effective. For AF or flutter with anomalous A-V conduction (*see* Case 175), any drug that blocks the conduction via an accessory pathway should be used. Under this circumstance quinidine or procainamide is very effective. Recently amiodarone was found to be extremely effective for all kinds of tachyarrhythmias associated with WPW syndrome.

When the conventional drug therapy is ineffective, EPS should be performed for possible cardiac surgery in selected cases.

Customarily WPW syndrome is classified into two types, depending upon the direction of the delta waves.

Type A:
The QRS complexes are primarily positive (upright) in lead V_1 (often all precordial leads) because the delta waves are directed anteriorly.

Type B:
The QRS complexes are primarily negative (downward) in lead V_1 (at times in leads V_{1-3}) because the delta waves are directed posteriorly and to the left.

Type A WPW syndrome superficially resembles RBBB, RVH, and posterior MI. Conversely, type B WPW syndrome (*see* Case 169) mimics LBBB, anteroseptal MI, and LVH. In both types diaphragmatic MI may be closely simulated (pseudodiaphragmatic MI) because the delta waves are often directed superiorly, as seen in this case.

This patient's WPW syndrome belongs to type A.

A routine ECG tracing was obtained from a 61-year-old man. He was found to be healthy, although his ECG finding is definitely abnormal.

    1. What is the ECG diagnosis?

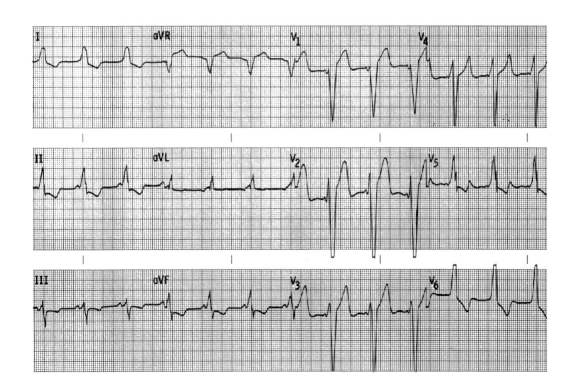

Diagnosis

The cardiac rhythm is sinus, with a rate of 72 beats per minute.

The ECG finding closely mimics LBBB because of broad QRS complexes that are primarily negative in leads V_{1-4} and upright in leads V_{5-6}, with secondary T wave change. Upon close observation, however, the diagnosis of WPW syndrome, type B, can be entertained using the conventional criteria (*see* Case 168). Note that the PR interval is short and the QRS complex is broad as a result of the delta wave. The initial slurring (delta wave) of the QRS complexes is observed because of the premature activation of a portion of the ventricles via an anomalous conduction.

This ECG tracing was obtained from a 26-year-old healthy female. She was referred to a cardiac clinic because her ECG was found to be abnormal.

    1. What is the ECG diagnosis?

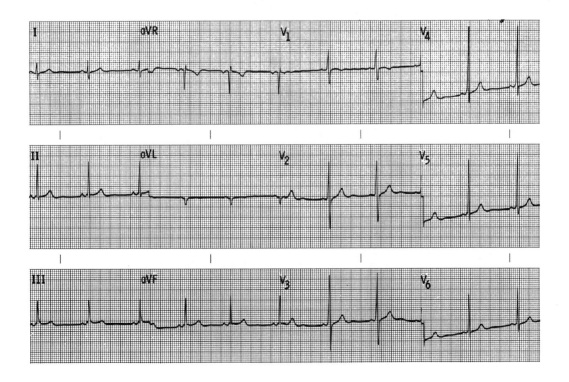

Diagnosis

The cardiac rhythm is sinus arrhythmia, with a rate of 63 beats per minute.

At a glance the patient's ECG appears to be normal, especially to inexperienced readers. Upon close observation, however, the diagnosis of WPW syndrome, type A, can be made using the conventional criteria (*see* Case 168).

In some cases of WPW syndrome the QRS complex may be extremely broad (*see* Case 169), whereas other cases (like this patient) may show only slightly prolonged QRS complex, depending upon the duration of the delta wave. By and large the delta wave is less pronounced when the accessory pathway is located very near to the normal A-V conduction system.

No further diagnostic test is necessary as long as the individual is asymptomatic. Likewise, no treatment is indicated for asymptomatic WPW syndrome.

This ECG tracing, obtained from a 71-year-old woman, was discussed during a weekly ECG conference.

1. What is the ECG diagnosis?

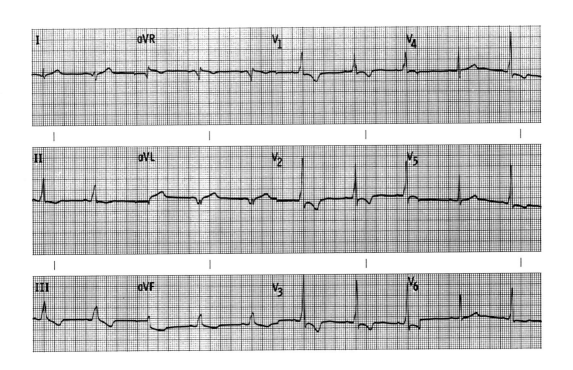

Diagnosis

The cardiac rhythm is sinus, with a rate of 60 beats per minute.

Upon a close observation many readers should be able to recognize that the configuration of the QRS complexes varies, namely, there is intermittent WPW syndrome, type A. The second beat from the last is a normally conducted beat. In addition the configuration of the QRS com-plexes varies in some beats because of ventricular fusion beats of varying degrees. In other words, the degree of the cardiac impulse conduction via the accessory pathway and the normal A-V conduction system varies from time to time leading to varying QRS configurations. This finding is not uncommon.

A 53-year-old man with known WPW syndrome developed palpitations, and he has had similar episodes on many occasions in the past. He was *not* taking any medication on a regular basis, however.

1. What is the cardiac rhythm diagnosis?
2. What is the proper way of handling this patient?

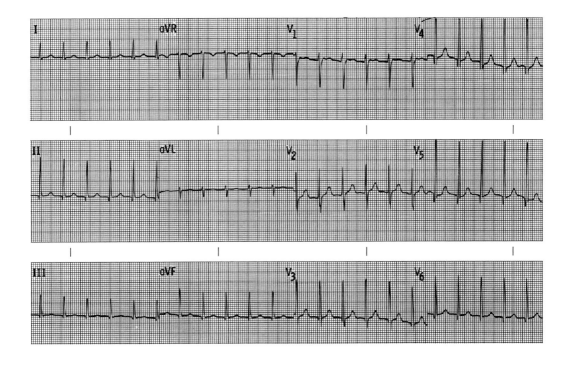

Diagnosis

The cardiac cycle is precisely regular, with no discernible P waves, and the QRS complexes are normal. This arrhythmia is often called supraventricular tachycardia without specifying the exact origin of the tachycardia. When this type of tachyarrhythmia occurs in WPW syndrome, the term "reciprocating tachycardia" (re-entrant tachycardia) is used because the tachycardia under this circumstance is considered to be due to the re-entry mechanism.

The drugs that may be very effective in preventing or terminating reciprocating tachycardia with normal QRS complexes include beta blockers (eg, propranolol), digoxin, and calcium blockers (eg, vera-pamil). When the QRS complexes are broad because of anomalous A-V conduction, the above-mentioned drugs are ineffective. Quinidine or quinidine-like drugs (eg, procainamide) are effective for broad QRS tachycardia in WPW syndrome. Amiodarone is found to be very effective for all kinds of tachyarrhythmia in WPW syndrome.

CSS is often effective in terminating reciprocating tachycardia in WPW syndrome. When the clinical situation is extremely urgent because of a very rapid rate, DC shock should be applied immediately. EPS is performed only for patients with refractory tachyarrhythmias in WPW syndrome.

This ECG tracing, taken on a 62-year-old man, was discussed during a weekly advanced ECG conference.

1. What is the ECG diagnosis?

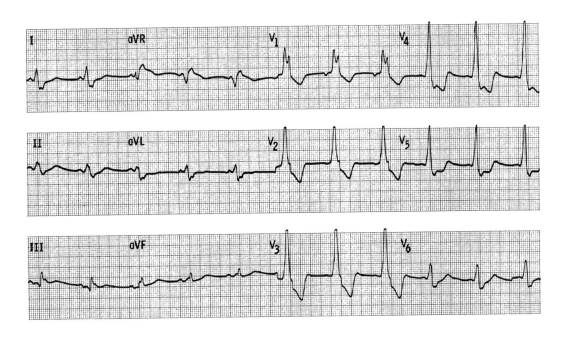

Diagnosis

The cardiac rhythm is sinus, with a rate of 64 beats per minute.

The QRS complexes are extremely broad because of two combined factors, namely, the diagnosis of RBBB can be readily made by all readers using the conventional criteria (see Case 34). However, the coexisting WPW syndrome, type A may *not* be recognized by most inexperienced readers.

It should be remembered that WPW syndrome causes the initial slurring (delta wave) of the QRS complexes, whereas the terminal portion of the QRS complexes is slurred by RBBB.

Coexisting RBBB with WPW syndrome is a very rare occurrence.

A 24-year-old apparently healthy man was referred to a cardiologist for evaluation of frequent rapid heart actions. The Holter monitor ECG was obtained to determine the nature of the paroxysmal rapid heart actions. The patient's 12-lead ECG was entirely within normal limits (not shown here).

1. What is the ECG diagnosis?

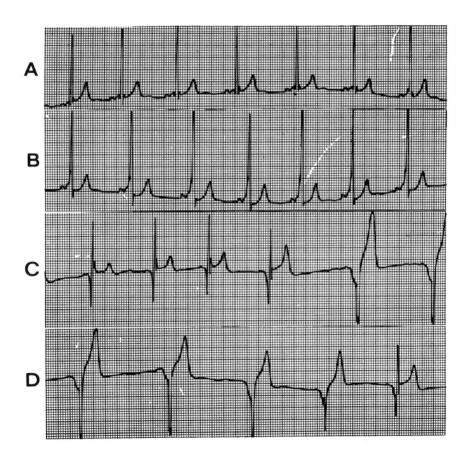

Diagnosis

The rhythm strips **A** through **D** are not continuous. The Holter monitor ECG reveals sinus arrhythmia with periods of marked sinus bradycardia (rate: 42–57 beats per minute). Unfortunately no episode of the paroxysmal rapid heart action was recorded on the Holter monitor ECG. The most interesting finding, however, was the WPW syndrome, with multiple anomalous A-V conductions causing various QRS complex configurations.

Later a paroxysmal supraventricular (reciprocating) tachycardia was documented on this patient by repeating the Holter monitor ECG (not shown here).

CASE 175

A 24-year-old healthy man developed rapid heart action; he had suffered from similar episodes previously. He was *not* taking any drugs.

1. What is the cardiac rhythm diagnosis during the rapid heart action?

2. What is the disorder underlying this rapid heart action?
3. What is the treatment of choice?

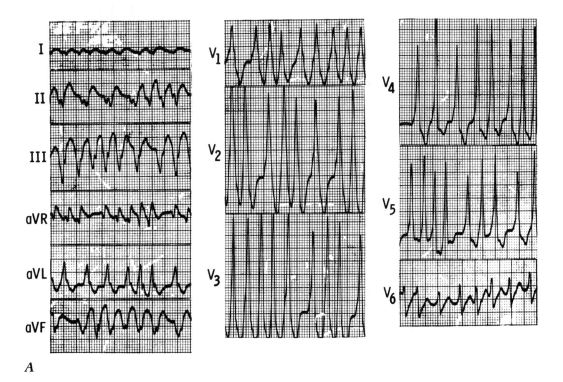

A

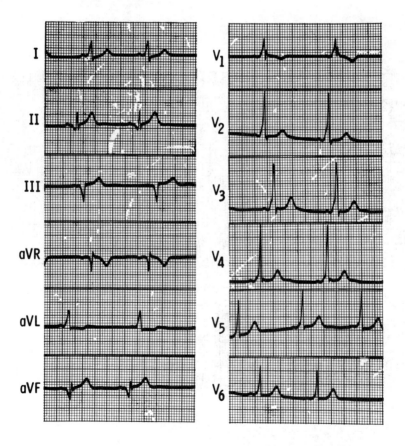

I
II
III
aVR
aVL
aVF

V₁
V₂
V₃
V₄
V₅
V₆

B

Diagnosis

12-lead ECG (during paroxysm):
The cardiac rhythm appears to be VT or even VF. However, the correct diagnosis is AF with anomalous A-V conduction due to the WPW syndrome, type A. The ventricular rate is extremely rapid (180–300 beats per minute), and the QRS configuration is broad and bizarre. The diagnosis of the WPW syndrome, type A is obvious during sinus rhythm.

The therapeutic approach to various tachyarrhythmias in WPW syndrome has been described previously (*see* Cases 168 and 172). By and large AF with anomalous A-V conduction, as seen in this case, is much more difficult to manage as compared to reciprocating tachycardia. Because of extremely rapid ventricular rate in AF under this circumstance, immediate application of DC shock is highly recommended before using any medication. Long-term drug therapy is indicated following termination of AF in WPW syndrome in most cases to prevent recurrence of the tachyarrhythmia. EPS is indicated for refractory cases for possible surgical consideration.

12-lead ECG (after paroxysm):
The cardiac rhythm appears to be VT or even VF. The diagnosis of the WPW syndrome, type A is obvious (*see* Case 168). Note a pseudodiaphragmatic and posterior MI pattern during sinus rhythm because of the type A WPW syndrome.

CHAPTER TEN

UNCOMMON ARRHYTHMIAS

CASE 176

This ECG tracing was obtained from a 71-year-old man.

1. What is the cardiac rhythm diagnosis?

2. What is the clinical significance of this arrhythmia?

3. What is the ECG diagnosis?

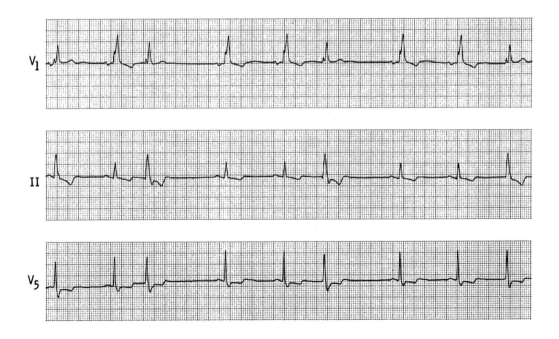

Diagnosis

The underlying cardiac rhythm is sinus bradycardia, with a rate of 56 beats per minute.

There are four ventricular ectopic beats that appear to be VPCs. Upon close observation, however, these ventricular ectopies are found to be not ordinary VPCs, namely, the coupling intervals vary, and the shortest interectopic intervals remain constant. Thus the diagnosis of ventricular parasystole is entertained.

Diagnostic Criteria of Parasystole

- Varying coupling intervals.
- Constant shortest interectopic intervals.
- Long interectopic intervals are multiples of the shortest interectopic intervals.
- Occasional fusion beats (not always present).

Clinically parasystole is a benign cardiac arrhythmia and is self-limited. Ventricular parasystole is the commonest occurrence, and atrial or A-V junctional parasystole is relatively uncommon (see Cases 177, 178, 181 and 182). The usual heart rates of parasystole range from 30–50 beats per minute.

The diagnosis of RBBB is obvious (see Case 34).

CASE 177

This ECG tracing, taken on a 74-year-old woman, was discussed during a weekly ECG conference.

    1. What is the cardiac rhythm diagnosis?

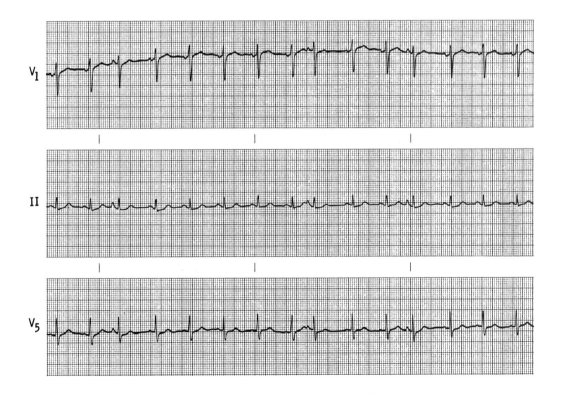

Diagnosis

The underlying cardiac rhythm is sinus rhythm, with a rate of 92 beats per minute. There are three atrial ectopic beats (the 3rd, 9th, and 12th beats) that show varying coupling intervals with constant, shortest, interectopic intervals. Thus the diagnosis of atrial parasystole (rate: 33 beats per minute) is made.

The diagnostic criteria of parasystole have been described previously (see Case 176).

This ECG tracing was taken on a 77-year-old man.

1. What is the cardiac rhythm diagnosis?

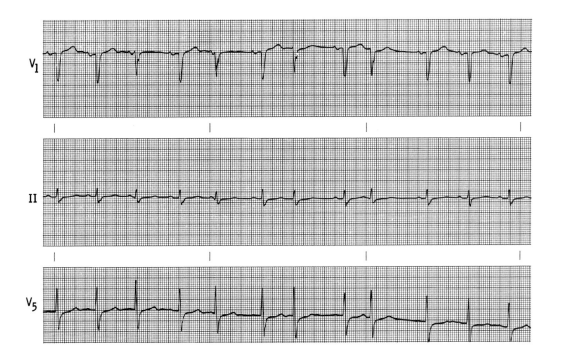

Diagnosis

The underlying cardiac rhythm is sinus, with a rate of 75 beats per minute.

The diagnosis of A-V junctional parasystole (rate: 40 beats per minute) can be established using the conventional criteria (*see* Case 176). The QRS complexes of the parasystolic beats (the 3rd, 5th, 7th, and 9th beats) are slightly deformed because of aberrant ventricular conduction. An alternative diagnosis is ventricular parasystole (arising from around the ventricular septum), judging from the slightly deformed parasystolic beats.

This ECG tracing, obtained from a 58-year-old man, was discussed during a weekly arrhythmia conference.

1. What is the cardiac rhythm diagnosis?

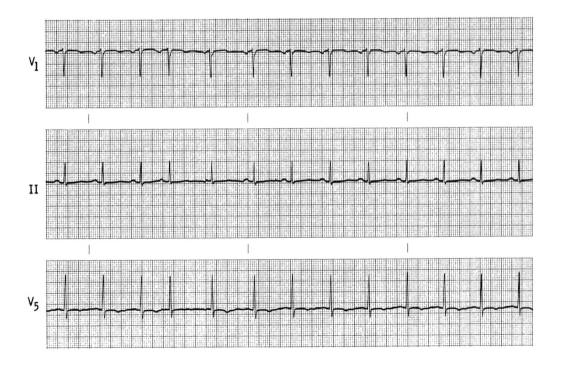

V_1

II

V_5

Diagnosis

The underlying cardiac rhythm is sinus, with a rate of 84 beats per minute. There is an atrial premature contraction (APC, the fourth beat), and the P wave of the sinus beat (the fifth beat) immediately following an APC is deformed. This deformed sinus P wave is termed "aberrant atrial conduction" (Chung's phenomenon).

Aberrant atrial conduction is considered to occur because of the alteration of the refractory period in the atria following an APC. Aberrant atrial conduction is insignificant clinically, but the ECG finding may mimic A-V JEBs or atrial escape beats.

DI was suspected in a 70-year-old woman with chronic advanced CHF.

1. What is the cardiac rhythm diagnosis?

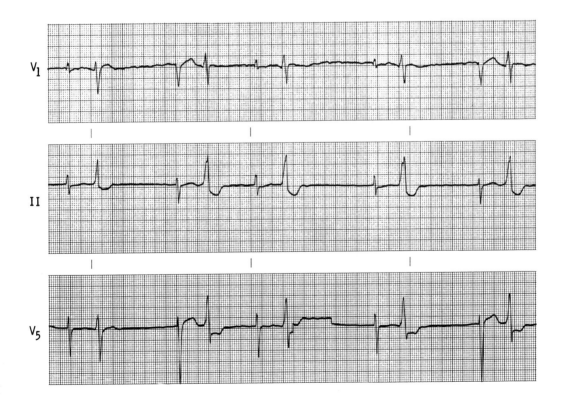

Diagnosis

The underlying cardiac rhythm is AF, but the ventricular rate is very slow (rate: 45–55 beats per minute) because of advanced A-V block. In addition there are occasional VEBs (the third and ninth beats), again as a result of advanced A-V block.

There are many bizarre beats that represent frequent multifocal VPCs, producing ventricular bigeminy.

When dealing with the above-mentioned arrhythmia, the underlying cause is almost always advanced DI.

CASE 181

This ECG tracing, obtained from a 55-year-old man, was presented to the weekly arrhythmia conference.

1. What is the cardiac rhythm diagnosis?
2. What is the ECG diagnosis?

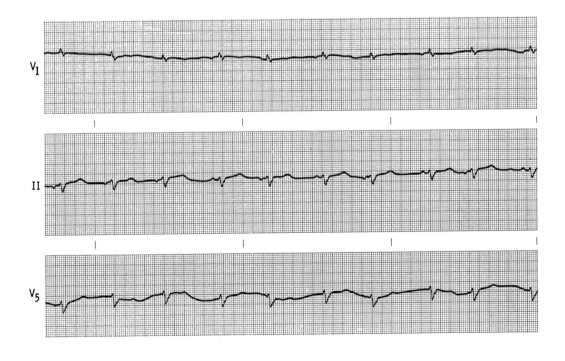

Diagnosis

The underlying cardiac rhythm is sinus, but there are frequent ectopic P waves that are conducted to the atria in a retrograde fashion. The ectopic rhythm represents A-V junctional parasystole, with a rate of 57 beats per minute. The diagnostic criteria of parasystole are found elsewhere (*see* Case 176).

There are only four sinus beats (the fourth, sixth, eighth, and tenth beats), and the remaining beats are A-V junctional parasystolic beats.

The diagnosis of BFB, which consists of RBBB and left anterior hemiblock, can be established using the conventional criteria (*see* Case 7).

This ECG tracing was taken on a 67-year-old woman with no demonstrable heart disease.

1. What is the cardiac rhythm diagnosis?

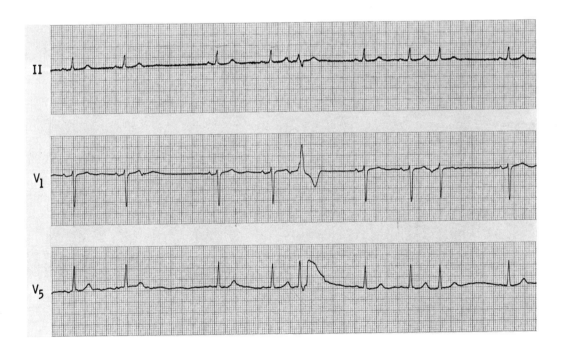

Diagnosis

The underlying cardiac rhythm is sinus (rate: 63 beats per minute), but there are three ectopic P waves. It is interesting to note that the first ectopic P wave (the third beat) is *not* conducted to the ventricles, whereas the second ectopic P wave is followed by a bizarre QRS complex because of aberrant ventricular conduction (the sixth beat). The last ectopic P wave is normally conducted to the ventricles (the ninth beat).

When the conventional criteria of parasystole (*see* Case 176) are utilized, the diagnosis of atrial parasystole (rate: 33 beats per minute) can be made without any difficulty.

This ECG tracing, obtained from a 29-year-old apparently healthy man, was discussed during a weekly advanced arrhythmia conference.

1. What is the cardiac rhythm diagnosis?

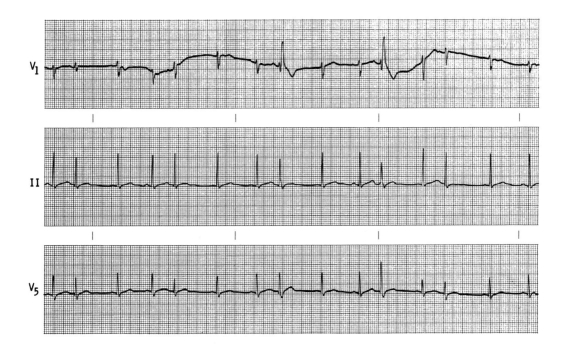

Diagnosis

The underlying cardiac rhythm is sinus (rate: 80 beats per minute), but there are frequent APCs producing atrial bigeminy and trigeminy. It is interesting to observe that all APCs are followed by deformed QRS complexes of varying degrees. This finding indicates aberrant ventricular conduction of varying degrees (*see* Case 98).

Some experienced readers should be able to recognize that the sinus P waves immediately following the APCs are deformed. This rare ECG finding represents aberrant atrial conduction (Chung's phenomenon), which has been described in detail earlier (*see* Case 179).

This ECG tracing was taken on a 28-year-old woman with mild hypertension. Because of her unusual P wave configuration, this ECG was presented to the weekly arrhythmia conference.

1. What is the cardiac rhythm diagnosis?

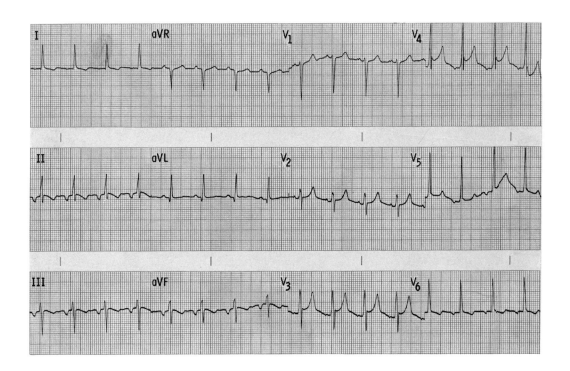

Diagnosis

The P waves are definitely abnormal because they are inverted in leads II, III, aVF, and V_{4-6} and upright in leads aVR, aVL, and V_{1-2}. Thus these ECG findings represent retrograde atrial activation. From a vectorial approach the P axis is directed superiorly and anteriorly, and the P wave vector is moving away from the left atrium. When these findings are interpreted carefully, the origin of the ectopic P waves can be determined, namely, the cardiac rhythm represents left atrial rhythm, with a rate of 94 beats per minute.

Characteristic Features of Left Atrial Rhythm

- Only upright (positive) component of P wave in lead V_1.
- Inverted P waves in inferior leads.
- Inverted P waves in leads V_{4-6}.
- Inverted (or biphasic) P wave in lead I.

The clinical significance of left atrial rhythm is uncertain, but this arrhythmia may be found in patients with left atrial enlargement.

This ECG tracing was obtained from a 76-year-old woman with possible DI.

1. What is the cardiac rhythm diagnosis?
2. What is the best therapeutic approach?

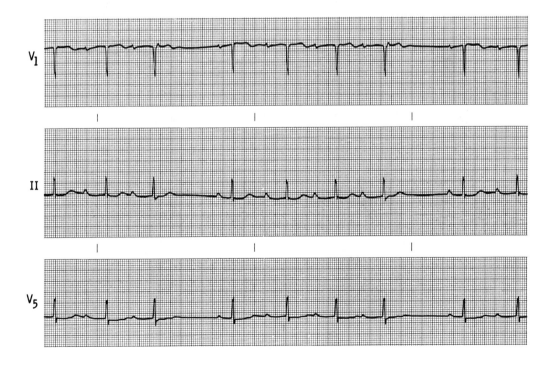

V_1

II

V_5

Diagnosis

The underlying cardiac rhythm is sinus (atrial rate: 65 beats per minute), with Wenckebach A-V block (A-V conduction ratio: 5 : 4). The characteristic features of Wenckebach A-V block are altered by a retrograde P wave following the QRS complex with the longest PR interval. Because of the retrograde P wave, the expected blocked sinus P wave fails to occur during Wenckebach A-V block. The retrograde P wave following the QRS complex with the longest PR interval is due to a re-entry phenomenon that occurs in the A-V junction.

This retrograde P wave represents a blocked reciprocal beat or atrial echo beat. The retrograde P wave (atrial echo beat) is superimposed to the end portion of the QRS complex so that inexperienced readers may fail to recognize it.

Discontinuation of digitalis is usually sufficient to treat mild digitalis-induced arrhythmias such as Wenckebach A-V block as long as the ventricular rate is reasonably fast (not slower than 45 beats per minute) and the patient is asymptomatic from the arrhythmia itself.

These ECG tracings, obtained from a 52-year-old man with a known COPD, were discussed during a weekly advanced ECG conference. Tracing **A** represents his 12-lead ECG, whereas tracing **B** is his cardiac rhythm strips.

1. What is the ECG diagnosis?
2. What is the clinical significance of this ECG abnormality?

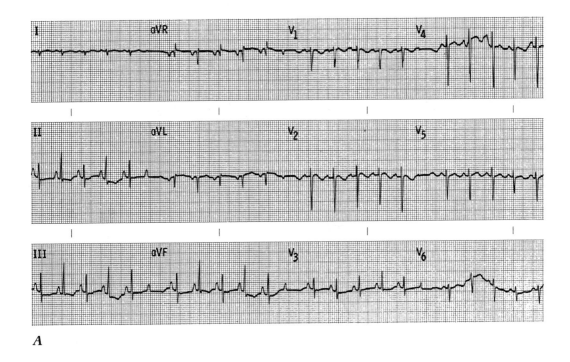

A

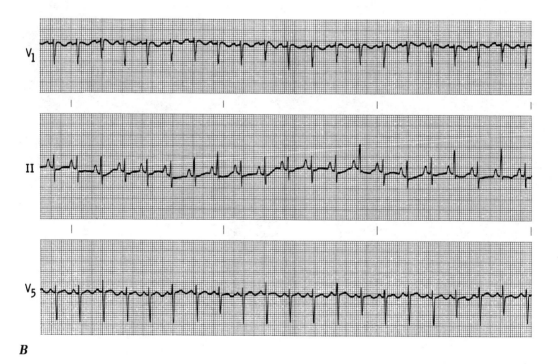

B

Diagnosis

The cardiac rhythm is sinus tachycardia, with a rate of 130 beats per minute. It is interesting to note that the configuration of the QRS complexes alters on every other beat in most areas. This ECG finding is termed "electrical alternans," which involves most commonly the QRS complexes.

The term "ventricular electrical alternans" is used when the electrical alternans involves only QRS complexes. The alternating ratio is most commonly 2 : 1, as seen in this case. Less commonly the 3 : 1 or 4 : 1 electrical alternans may be observed.

Rarely the electrical alternans may involve the P waves, the ST segment, and the T waves. By and large ventricular electrical alternans is often associated with electrical alternans involving the ST segment and T waves, as seen in this case.

The commonest underlying disorders in the production of electrical alternans include advanced CHF and pericardial effusion (see Case 200).

The diagnosis of P-pulmonale and RVH are strongly considered (see Case 45).

CHAPTER ELEVEN

MISCELLANEOUS ARRHYTHMIAS

This ECG tracing was taken on a 20-year-old man with advanced renal failure, and he was scheduled to have renal transplantation in the near future.

    1. What is the ECG diagnosis?

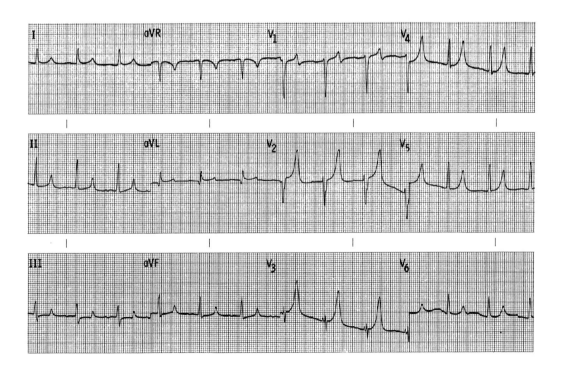

Diagnosis

The cardiac rhythm is sinus, with a rate of 70 beats per minute, and first degree A-V block.

There are two striking ECG abnormalities due to hyperkalemia and hypocalcemia as a result of advanced renal failure.

Hyperkalemia-induced ECG abnormalities include first degree A-V block and flat P waves associated with tent-shaped and tall T waves in many leads (*see* Case 94).

Prolonged QT interval as a result of the lengthening of the ST segment is a characteristic feature of hypocalcemia. In advanced renal failure hyperkalemia and hypocalcemia often coexist.

CASE 188

This ECG tracing was taken on a 65-year-old woman with DI.

1. What is the cardiac rhythm diagnosis?
2. What is the ECG diagnosis?

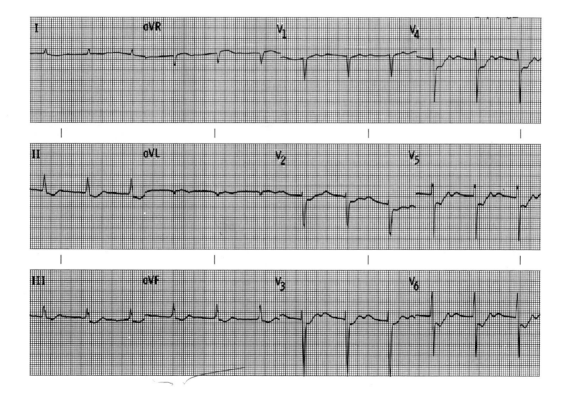

Diagnosis

The cardiac rhythm is nonparoxysmal A-V JT, with a rate of 72 beats per minute. The atrial mechanism is most likely AF, so that there is complete A-V dissociation. By reviewing her previous ECG tracings, she was found to have chronic AF for several years in the past.

There are prominent U waves in all precordial leads, indicative of hypokalemia (*see* Case 95). It has been shown that hypokalemia predisposes to DI.

The ST segment depression (horizontal to downsloping) in many leads is strongly suggestive of diffuse subendocardial injury, although digitalis effect may be partially responsible for this finding.

CASE 189

This ECG tracing, which belongs to a 33-year-old man, was presented to the weekly ECG conference without any clinical information.

    1. What is the ECG diagnosis?

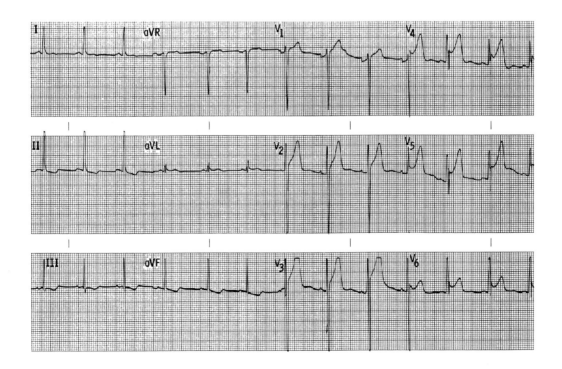

Diagnosis

The cardiac rhythm is sinus, with a rate of 68 beats per minute.

It is easy to recognize that the ST segment is elevated in leads V_{2-6}, primarily as a result of "J"-point elevation. This ECG finding is commonly found in healthy black males, and the term "early repolarization pattern" is used under this circumstance.

When the early repolarization pattern is pronounced, the ECG finding may simulate acute pericarditis or hypothermia-induced ECG abnormality.

LVH and left atrial enlargement are strongly considered (see Cases 10 and 33).

CASE 190

A 26-year-old man was examined in the ER
for the evaluation of his chest pain.

1. What is the ECG diagnosis?

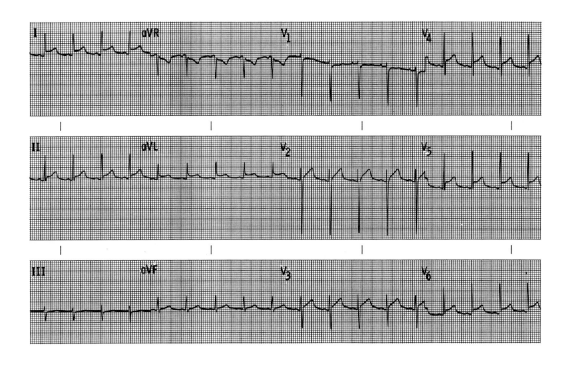

Diagnosis

The cardiac rhythm is sinus tachycardia, with a rate of 106 beats per minute.

It should be noted that the ST segment is elevated in many leads diffusely. This ECG abnormality is a characteristic feature of acute pericarditis. He was proven to have acute viral pericarditis. Remember that a pure pericarditis produces diffuse ST segment elevation involving practically every lead, but abnormal Q waves never occur.

When pericarditis becomes subacute and chronic, the ST segment returns to the baseline, but inverted T waves occur in many leads.

CASE 191

This ECG tracing was obtained from a 65-year-old woman with a permanent artificial pacemaker. She was not taking any medication.

1. What is the cardiac rhythm diagnosis?
2. What is the mechanism responsible for the production of the prematurely occurring beats?

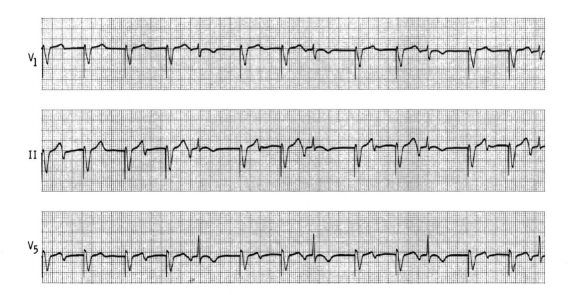

Diagnosis

The cardiac rhythm is an artificial pace-maker-induced ventricular rhythm with Wenckebach ventriculoatrial block and frequent reciprocal beats that occur on every third beat. It should be noted that the RP intervals progressively lengthen because of Wenckebach ventriculoatrial block, but the reciprocal beat occurs following the longest RP interval.

Of course the reciprocal beats occur as a result of the re-entry phenomenon in the A-V junction. The re-entry phenomenon tends to occur when there is marked depression of the conductivity in the A-V junction, especially when there is the depression of unequal degrees in the A-V junction. The artificial pacemaker function is normal in this case.

CASE 192

This ECG tracing was obtained from a hypertensive 51-year-old woman with a cerebrovascular accident.

1. What is the ECG diagnosis?

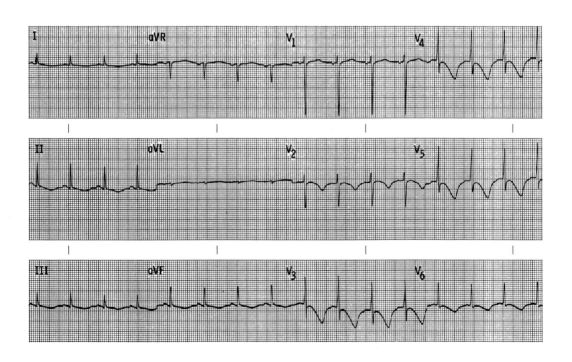

Diagnosis

The cardiac rhythm is sinus, with a rate of 90 beats per minute.

It is obvious that the T waves are inverted in many leads, and the QT interval is markedly prolonged because of broad T wave. This ECG finding is often observed in patients with a variety of CNS disorders. The exact underlying mechanism responsible for the production of this T wave abnormality in CNS disorders is *not* clearly understood.

The ECG finding in various CNS disorders may closely simulate other clinical conditions, including pericarditis, myocarditis, and myocardial ischemia.

In addition LVH is considered (*see* Case 10).

This ECG tracing was obtained from a healthy 21-year-old female.

  1. What is the ECG diagnosis?

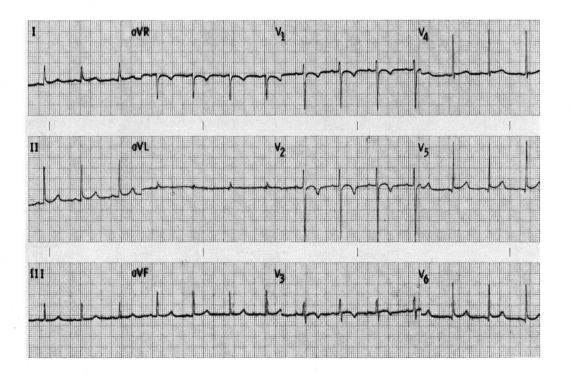

Diagnosis

The cardiac rhythm is sinus arrhythmia, with a rate of 82 beats per minute.

At a glance the ECG appears to be abnormal because T waves are inverted in leads V_{1-3}. However, most experienced readers should be able to diagnose the "juvenile T wave pattern," which is a normal variant.

The juvenile T wave pattern is much commoner among healthy young women than in males. This ECG pattern gradually disappears as the individual gets older.

The juvenile T wave pattern is almost a rule rather than an exception in children and many young adults (younger than 20 years). This normal variant is rather unusual in individuals older than 30 years.

When dealing with inverted T waves, the ECG finding superficially simulates other clinical conditions such as myocardial ischemia, pericarditis, or myocarditis. By and large the T wave inversion in the juvenile T wave pattern is *not* deep and is *not* symmetric.

CASE 194

This ECG tracing, obtained from a 49-year-old man with prostate cancer, was discussed during a weekly ECG conference.

1. What is the ECG diagnosis?

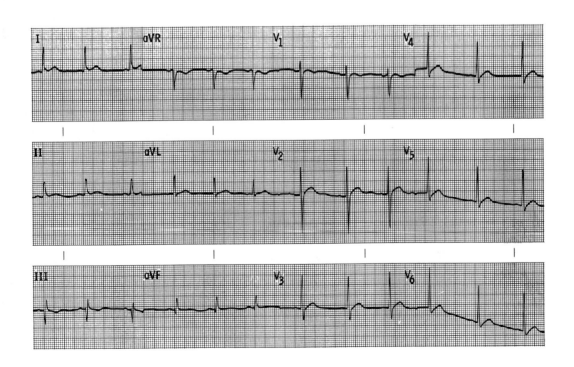

Diagnosis

The cardiac rhythm is sinus arrhythmia, with a rate of 62–75 beats per minute.

The striking ECG abnormality in this tracing is markedly shortened QT interval. The QT interval is very short, primarily because the ST segment is practically absent. This unique ECG abnormality is a characteristic feature of hypercalcemia.

This patient was found to have a markedly elevated calcium level in the blood as a result of bone metastasis from his prostate carcinoma. There is no other situation causing marked shortening of the QT interval besides hypercalcemia.

CASE 195

A 21-year-old man underwent open heart surgery for removal of a diverticulum from the left ventricle. This ECG tracing was taken soon after the cardiac surgery.

1. What is the ECG abnormality?

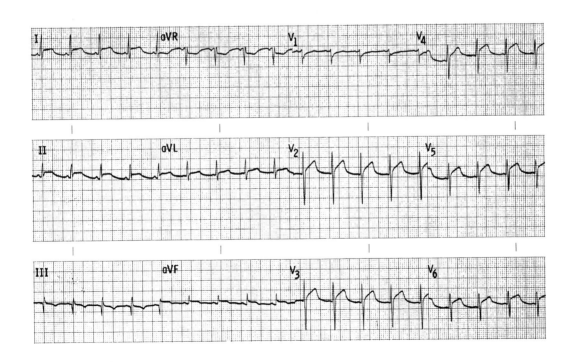

Diagnosis

The cardiac rhythm is sinus tachycardia, with a rate of 102 beats per minute.

It should be noted that the ST segment is diffusely elevated in practically all leads. This ECG abnormality is a characteristic feature of acute pericarditis (see Case 190). The ECG finding in acute pericarditis is identical, regardless of the underlying cause (eg, viral, traumatic, or postsurgical).

Later the ST segment elevation is followed by inverted T waves, again involving many ECG leads when pericarditis becomes more than a few days old. In acute pericarditis the ECG finding closely mimics an early sign of acute MI before pathologic Q waves are fully produced.

A possibility of diaphragmatic MI is raised because of a deep Q wave in lead III.

This ECG tracing was taken following mitral as well as aortic valve replacement for advanced rheumatic heart disease.

1. What is the ECG diagnosis?

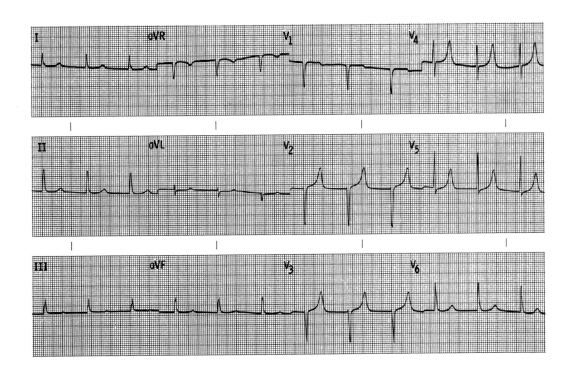

Diagnosis

The ventricular cycle is regular, with no discernible P waves. Thus the cardiac rhythm is nonparoxysmal A-V JT, with a rate of 68 beats per minute.

Most readers should be able to recognize tent-shaped and tall T waves involving many leads. This ECG finding indicates hyperkalemia.

Another ECG abnormality is prolonged QT interval, primarily due to lengthening of the ST segment. This ECG finding is due to hypocalcemia.

Therefore this ECG tracing demonstrates a combination of hyperkalemia and hypocalcemia (see Cases 94 and 187), which often occurs in patients with renal failure. This patient developed acute renal failure soon after the open cardiac surgery.

CASE 197

This ECG tracing, which was obtained from a 42-year-old hypertensive woman, was presented to a weekly ECG conference as an *unknown ECG*.

1. What is the ECG diagnosis?

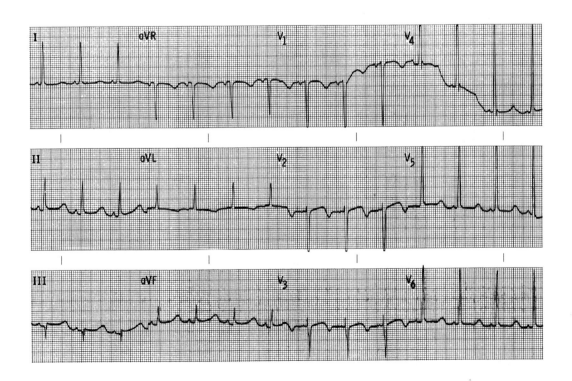

Diagnosis

The cardiac rhythm is sinus, with a rate of 80 beats per minute.

The striking ECG abnormality in this tracing is markedly prolonged QT interval as a result of lengthening of the ST segment. This ECG finding is a characteristic feature of hypocalcemia (*see* Cases 187 and 196). The duration of the T wave is *not* altered by hypocalcemia.

In addition the diagnosis of LVH is made using the conventional criteria (*see* Case 10).

CASE 198

A 23-year-old woman was examined at the cardiac clinic because of a heart murmur. A congenital heart disease was suspected.

1. What is the ECG diagnosis?
2. What is most likely the underlying congenital cardiac defect?

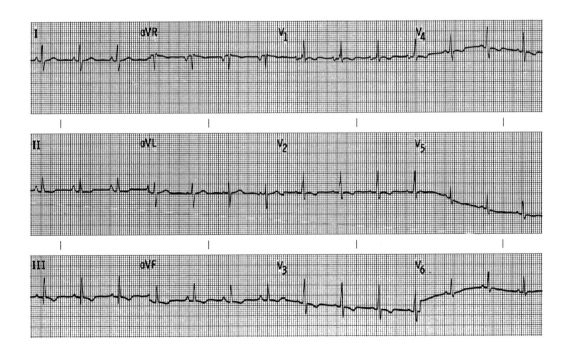

Diagnosis

The cardiac rhythm is sinus, with a rate of 80 beats per minute.

The diagnosis of incomplete RBBB can be established using the conventional criteria (*see* Case 34). Among all types of congenital heart diseases, atrial septal defect is most commonly associated with incomplete RBBB. Complete RBBB is less common in atrial septal defect.

Other congenital cardiac defects that are often associated with RBBB include tetralogy of Fallot, ventricular septal defect, and Ebstein's anomaly.

The P waves are slightly peaked in leads II and aVF, suggestive of RAH (*see* Case 45). The term "P-congenitale" is used to describe right atrial enlargement due to a variety of congenital heart diseases.

Pulmonary embolism was suspected in a 78-year-old man who was brought to the ER because of severe chest pain and marked dyspnea.

   1. What is the ECG diagnosis?

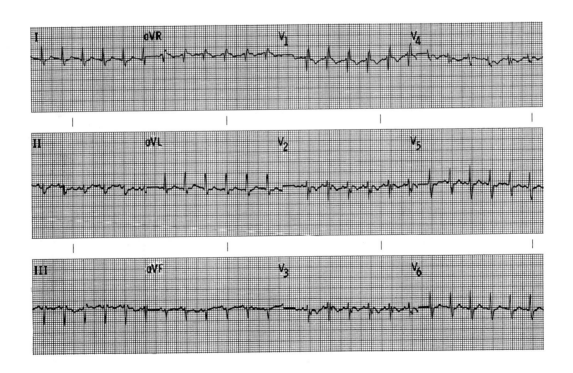

Diagnosis

The cardiac rhythm is marked sinus tachycardia, with a rate of 150 beats per minute.

The diagnosis of incomplete RBBB can be made using the conventional criteria (*see* Case 34). Another ECG abnormality is left anterior hemiblock (*see* Case 27). Thus the diagnosis of BFB is entertained (*see* Case 7).

Pulmonary embolism should be the first diagnostic consideration when any individual develops marked sinus tachycardia or atrial tachyarrhythmias associated with RBBB (complete or incomplete), especially when the diagnosis of acute MI is reasonably excluded. Other ECG abnormalities due to pulmonary embolism have been described previously (*see* Case 131).

Cardiac consultation was requested for the evaluation of an unusual ECG finding in a 36-year-old woman with advanced renal failure. She was not taking any cardiac drug.

1. What is the ECG abnormality?
2. What is the best therapeutic approach?

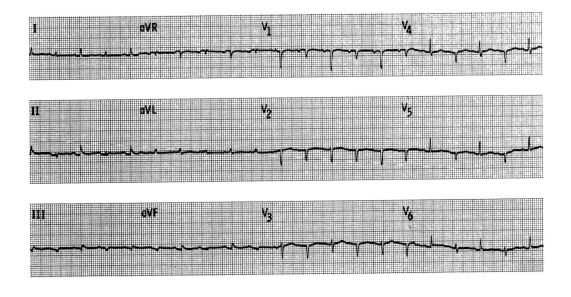

Diagnosis

The cardiac rhythm is sinus tachycardia, with a rate of 122 beats per minute. It is easily recognized that the QRS complex configurations change on every other beat. Thus the ECG abnormality is 2:1 ventricular electrical alternans.

Electrical alternans is most commonly observed in patients with massive pericardial effusion and/or severe CHF. Needless to say, massive pericardial effusion as a complication of uremic pericarditis was responsible for the production of electrical alternans in this patient. Pericardiocentesis was recommended as cardiac consultation.

Two to one electrical alternans (changing configuration on every other beat) is the commonest form of this entity. Any other alternating ratios, such as 3:1 electrical alternans, are only rarely observed.

Old diaphragmatic MI is strongly considered.

SUGGESTED READINGS

Chung EK: *Ambulatory Electrocardiography: Holter Monitor Electrocardiography.* New York: Springer-Verlag, 1979.

Chung EK: *Artificial Cardiac Pacing, ed 2.* Baltimore, Williams & Wilkins, 1984.

Chung EK: *A Clinical Manual of Cardiovascular Medicine.* Norwalk, CT, Appleton-Century-Crofts, 1984.

Chung EK: *Office Electrocardiography.* Baltimore, University Park Press, 1984.

Chung EK: *Principles of Cardiac Arrhythmias, ed 4.* Baltimore, Williams & Wilkins, 1987.

Chung EK: *Quick Reference to Cardiovascular Disease, ed 3.* Baltimore, Williams & Wilkins, 1987.

Chung EK, Chung LW: *Introduction to Clinical Cardiology.* Basel, Switzerland, S. Karger, 1983.

Chung EK: *Manual of Cardiac Arrhythmias.* New York, York Medical Books, 1986.

Chung EK: *Electrocardiography: Practical Applications With Vectorial Principles, ed 3.* Norwalk, CT, Appleton-Century-Crofts, 1985.

Fox W, Stein E: *Cardiac Rhythm Disturbances, A Step-By-Step Approach.* Philadelphia, Lea & Febiger, 1983.

Josephson ME, Seides SF: *Clinical Cardiac Electrophysiology. Techniques and Interpretations.* Philadelphia, Lea & Febiger, 1979.

Marriott HJL: *Practical Electrocardiography, ed 7.* Baltimore, Williams & Wilkins, 1983.

Marriott HJL, Conover MHB: *Advanced Concepts in Arrhythmias.* St. Louis, Mosby, 1983.

Morganroth J, Horowitz, LN: *Sudden Cardiac Death.* New York, Grune & Stratton, 1985.

Schamroth L: *The Disorders of Cardiac Rhythm, ed 2.* Oxford, England, Blackwell Scientific, 1980.

Zipes DP, Jalife J: *Cardiac Electrophysiology and Arrhythmias.* New York, Grune & Stratton, 1985.

Page numbers in bold indicate major discussions of ECG diagnostic types and syndromes.

Atrial premature contraction (APC) (*cont.*)
blocked, 234, 284
nonconducted, 266
with aberrant ventricular conduction, 232,
250, 284
Atrial septal defect, 426
Atrial tachyarrhythmia, **352,** 428
Atrial tachycardia (AT), 254, 352
A-V block and, 286
paroxysmal, 236
Wenckebach A-V block and, 296, 304
Atrial trigeminy, 392
Atrioventricular (A-V) block, 222, 256
advanced, 120, 192, 226, 248, 386
complete, 182, 194, 198, 200, 202, 282
first-degree, 18, 222, 224, 322, 404
Mobitz type I, 174
Mobitz type II, 158, 174, 178, 192
Wenckebach, 174, 176, 186, 196, 207, 296,
304, 306
Wenckebach advanced, 184, 190, 192
Atrioventricular (A-V) conduction,
Wenckebach, 290, 350
Atrioventricular (A-V) dissociation (com-
plete), 182
AF with fascicular tachycardia and, 308
atrial flutter-fibrillation and, 200
atrial flutter and, 282
AT and VT and, 352
A-V JER and, 198, 202
chronic AF and, 406
LBBB and, 194
nonparoxysmal A-V JT and, 326
Atrioventricular (A-V) dissociation (in-
complete), 180, 184, 190, 322, 346, 354
Atrioventricular junctional escape beat (A-V
JEB), intermittent, 120
Atrioventricular junctional escape rhythm
(A-V JER), 198, 216, 316, 318, 324, 330
Atrioventricular junctional tachycardia (A-V
JT), 236, 254, 278
intermittent nonparoxysmal, 158
nonparoxysmal, **12,** 16, 314, **320,** 322, 324,
326, 328, **332,** 348, 406, 422
paroxysmal, **312**
with intermittent exit block, 332
Atrioventricular (A-V) junctional arrhythmia,
12
Atrioventricular (A-V) junctional parasystole,
382, 388

Atrioventricular (A-V) nodal block, 174, 180
Atrioventricular (A-V) node, diseased, 220,
318
A-V: *See* Atrioventricular

BBBB: *See* Bilateral bundle branch block
BFB: *See* Bifascicular block
Biatrial hypertrophy, 118
diagnostic criteria of, **102**
Bifascicular block (BFB), **16,** 56, 139, 200,
240, 428
incomplete RBBB and left anterior hemiblock, 308
intermittent, 156
RBBB and left anterior hemiblock in, 146,
152, 158, 202, 252, 254, 268, 388
RBBB and left posterior hemiblock in, 140
Bigeminal rhythm, **290,** 306
Bilateral bundle branch block (BBBB), 152
advanced, 140
diagnostic criteria of, **16**
incomplete, 16, 254
Biventricular hypertrophy, 130
diagnostic criteria of, **120**
Bizarre QRS complexes, **240,** 250, 258, 274,
292, 358, 373, 390
Blocked reciprocal beats, 266, 396

Cardiogenic shock, 10
Cardiomyopathy, 10, 102
Central nervous system disorders (CNS), 414
CHF: *See* Congestive heart failure
Chronic obstructive pulmonary disease
(COPD), 10, 93, 105, 117, 125, 231, 245,
259, 260, 273, 279, 280, 397
advanced, 98
Chung's phenomenon: *See* Aberrant atrial
conduction
CNS disorders: *See* Central nervous system
disorders
Congenital heart disease, 121
Congestive heart failure, 10, 101, 107, 271
advanced, 399
chronic, 157
secondary to systemic hypertension, 113
severe, 430